Neurosensory Divergence:
Autistic Languages

Neurosensory Divergence: Autistic Languages

A Roadmap to an Equitable Life for Autistic Children

Helen Daniel

authors
AND CO.

First published in Great Britain in 2023
by Authors & Co.
www.authorsandco.pub

ISBN 978-1-915771-41-4 (paperback)
ISBN 978-1-915771-42-1 (hardback)

Medical Disclaimer

This book contains general information about medications and treatments. The information is not advice, and should not be treated as such. Do not substitute this information for the medical advice of physicians. The information contained in this book is based on the personal and professional experiences of the author. Always consult your doctor for yours and your family's individual needs.

Book Buddy

The book buddy which sits alongside this book can help those who are dyslexic or those who prefer to read books in smaller sections.

This book buddy video:

- Gives clear multi-modal (including visual) information on important parts of the book
- Gives an overview of important sections in the book
- Gives more information on ideas where needed

Download the book buddy here:
www.outsidetheboxsensory.com/start-here

To my favourite ones.

I am so happy that our world is one of acceptance and belief. I love you so very much.

You are my reason.

CONTENTS

ACKNOWLEDGEMENTS

To Tom, Ben and all my family and friends who have supported me throughout this process.

To all the dedicated teachers, Learning Support Assistants, SENCOs and school staff who think outside the box to support autistic and neurodivergent children (you know who you are.)

To Mima Cornish, who helped me to build true confidence in myself and my abilities.

To Gem Kennedy, who coached me with compassion and enabled me to breathe life into my dreams.

To Emma While and the rewilding collective, who helped me find my neurodivergent sparkle.

To my tutors Luke, Jill, Stephen and Andy, who framed my thoughts in new and exciting ways and taught me so much.

To my editor and friend Rhiannon Morgan-Jones, who has supported me over the last four years and always challenged me to ensure my writing was robust and well-balanced.

To Abi, Deanne and the whole team at Authors and Co., who believed in my fight and helped me get the words out there in this book.

And most importantly, to all the neurodivergent children, young people and adults who have shared their experiences with me.

Is the Author Autistic?

The answer to this is not straightforward. Although I have been identified as having a neurodivergent profile, I am also part of multiple marginalised groups; this means that unpicking where my traits stem from is complex.

As a child, I often seemed to miss social cues; this meant I got into trouble socially when I talked over others or was deemed to *go on* about subjects that interested me. I had intense interests that I would hyperfocus on, and I often got lost in my own imagination. Yet in school, teachers constantly told me I lacked focus, even though I put massive effort into staying on task. I also found it difficult to 'fit in' socially and often felt like I was speaking a different language because the intention behind my words was so often misunderstood.

As an adult, I have found strategies that work for my neurodivergent profile. I now have a wonderful group of friends I feel comfortable with. Although I was described as *lacking in focus* at school, I now have several higher education qualifications because I found things to study that sparked my passion. I work for myself, which removes some of the challenges neurodivergent people face in a typical workplace.

I am a qualified teacher with many years of experience in teaching and childcare. I have worked as an autism trainer and as a mentor to neurodivergent children and young people. I also have a Master's in autism studies and qualifications in both reading and speech acquisition. It is no coincidence that I have taken such an interest in autism and neurodivergence in my career. I have dedicated time and effort towards working out what makes neurodivergent children tick, including reflecting on my childhood. Like so many neurodivergent people, I have had to tread my own path to get where I am.

Although my experiences as a neurodivergent person have helped shape my ideas for this book, it is the stories from all the amazing autistic children, young people and adults* reflecting on their childhood that have brought it to life.

*Where appropriate, the names of adults and children have been changed to protect their identity. In some cases, their connection to me has also been changed.

Disclaimer

This book may not resonate with your idea of your autistic profile or experiences. This is, of course, valid and fully respected. I discuss autism and neurosensory divergence based on my own experiences, the experiences of those closest to me, and on the information that has been shared with me over the years.

I have endeavoured to reference sources as fully as possible. In the case that any amendments need to be made, please contact me via my website.

PREFACE

Neurosensory Divergence: Autistic Languages is a fight song. It is the fight song of so many parents, teachers, professionals, and advocates[1] who want to see a change in the world for autistic children and young people. Autistic adults who look back on their childhoods and autistic children alike are unwavering in their message that things need to change – not the small, incremental changes currently taking place, but giant leaps that completely alter current thinking around autism. It has become my mission to be part of that change. I want to empower autistic families to come home to their own intuition and find strength in following a new path. Deep in our souls, we know that current systems and structures are not serving our autistic children. Many of us feel there must be another way.

Many families of autistic children say that navigating the current systems that are supposed to support families can feel like trudging through treacle. The language used

1   Weldon, R. (2020). My Autistic Fight Song.

to describe autistic children and the reports that follow them are heartbreaking in many cases. These reports include words such as *disorder, delay* and *deficit*. This language does not describe the vibrant and wonderful autistic children in my family or those I have taught or mentored. Often, though, those autistic children *are* worn down by the considerable burden to survive and thrive in situations that do not serve them. Not only that, but society also tells them that because they are struggling with 'expected' targets, they are somehow failing at being a human child. I dispute this in the most robust terms possible.

I believe that autistic children thrive in the 'unexpected' – outside-the-box ways that are often overlooked. What if autistic children are learning things we have no idea about? What if their brilliance is stifled by the need to conform to the expected? And what if their autistic gaze on unexpected elements within environments is one of their most wondrous parts? To address these questions, I will first describe how our current systems and structures are organised and then propose ways in which we might move forward into the future.

The pages of this book are filled with the experiences of autistic children and adults, alongside affirming and validating research. These stories and experiences have led me to believe that the missing part of the autistic picture is to be found in autistic sensory experiences. The way humans learn, live and express themselves all starts with our senses. Through our sensory experience of the world, we come to build concepts and beliefs, and autistic children are doing just that. But they inhabit a world that often fails to grasp their autistic 'ways of being'.

This book offers a new understanding of autism through a sensory lens called Neurosensory Divergence (NSD). Through this lens, it becomes evident that the communication, learning styles, and traits of many autistic children are intricately connected with their sensory access. Neurosensory Divergence positions as *natural, understandable and valid* an autistic child's responses to their sensory experiences. It also elevates sensory experiences within some autistic profiles as being *the* most important aspect when planning adjustments. Autistic traits have long been 'othered' and seen as inappropriate, leading to huge burdens of stigma and trauma for the autistic population.

Neurosensory Divergence: Autistic Languages does not negate the challenges autistic people face; I one hundred per cent acknowledge that having an autistic or neurodivergent profile makes life more challenging – I know, I have lived it, too! Instead, I want to lay bare the ways autistic children are often let down. I genuinely believe that a better understanding of autistic sensory profiles and internal processes can lead to greater understanding and better supports. This book discusses where we are now and how old ideas still shape current thinking. I explain how I came to form ideas around Neurosensory Divergence and how current practices often fail to support NSD fully. Finally, I lay out a road map for how we should do things differently when supporting autistic children through this new lens.

I have written this book to show that there *is* another way.

> '*Do the best you can until you know better. Then, when you know better, do better.*'

Maya Angelou

GLOSSARY

Language Choices

Child with autism *versus* **autistic child** The former term positions autism as a problem within the child.[2] I do not view autistic sensory experiences and traits as separate from the child but rather as an integral part[3] of them. Therefore, I will use the term *autistic child* throughout this book.

Equality *versus* **equity** *Equality* means each individual or group of people is given the same resources or opportunities. *Equity* recognises that everyone has different requirements and each person should be provided with the resources and opportunities they need to reach an equal outcome.

---

2   Kenny, L., Hattersley, C., Molins, B., Buckley, C., Povey, C. and Pellicano, E. (2016). Which terms should be used to describe autism? Perspectives from the UK autism community. Autism, 20(4), pp.442–462. doi:https://doi.org/10.1177/1362361315588200.

3   Anon, (n.d.). Why I dislike 'person first' language- Jim Sinclair | Autism MythBusters. [online] Available at: https://autismmyth busters.com/general-public/autistic-vs-people-with-autism/jim-sin clair-why-i-dislike-person-first-language/ [Accessed 13 Oct. 2022].

Behaviours *versus* **traits** Although the wording 'autistic traits' holds less stigma than behaviours, the terms are used interchangeably in this book to assist with its readability.

Challenging behaviours *versus* **behaviours that challenge others** When children are placed in situations that are not optimal for their profile, they may display behaviours that others around them find challenging. Changing the way we describe these behaviours from 'challenging behaviours' to 'behaviours which challenge others' moves those behaviours from being an integral part of the child to being a problem to be solved by those around them.

Non- or pre-verbal *versus* **non- or pre-speaking** The terms non-speaking and pre-speaking are used because autistic children may use verbalisation to convey meaning. Therefore, the term non-verbal is not appropriate.

Terms Used

Hyperfocus Autistic people are known to have the ability to focus intensely on subjects and activities that pique their interest.

Monotropic mind A tendency to hyperfocus for long periods on something of interest and process one sensory channel at a time.

Polytropic mind Having multiple interests aroused at any time, pulling in multiple strands of sensory information, both external and internal.

Hyper-polytropic mind This can feel like being pulled in multiple sensory directions at once.

Autistic 'ways of being' Autistic experiences and internal processes. These can be mental, physical or emotional factors, and impact how a person interacts in the world. Internal processes can give rise to ways of behaving or responding.

DSM-5 *(American Psychiatric Association [APA], 2013)* A manual for the assessment and diagnosis of mental disorders. This manual includes diagnostic criteria currently used to diagnose autism.

Special Educational Needs The term used to describe the need that children have to learn in ways other than that offered by a mainstream education. This includes children with diagnoses such as dyslexia, dyspraxia, ADHD, autism etc.

Spiky learning profile A learning profile in which strengths and weaknesses are more pronounced than the average. This means that a child might show abilities in specific areas of learning, such as maths, but might also experience challenges in other areas, such as handwriting or working memory.

Expected In England, set expectations are built on the concept that children should acquire skills at set ages. These abilities are perceived to be those of the average child. How a child is 'expected' to develop is built into health and education systems.

Divergence The difference between two or more things.

Neurodiversity The range of differences in brain function in the whole population. This refers to all people.

Neurodivergence Brain function which diverges from the average or expected. This term includes anyone whose brain functioning diverges, including those who are autistic, dyslexic and those with attention deficit hyperactivity disorder.

Neurosensory Divergence Brain and sensory function which diverges from the average or expected.

Sensory divergence Relates specifically to divergent sensory experiences. *Sensory divergence* is used instead of *sensory processing disorder* to remove the stigma currently associated with having a divergent sensory profile.

Sensory stimulus An event or object received by the senses that elicits a response.[4]

Stimming Repetitive movements or vocalisations

Scaffolding Support which develops a child's knowledge beyond their current point of learning.

Co-morbid conditions Medical conditions that present in a person simultaneously.

---

4   Lestrud, M. (2013). Sensory Stimuli. Encyclopedia of Autism Spectrum Disorders, [online] pp.2816–2817. doi:https://doi.org/10.1007/978-1-4419-1698-3_1597.

Body communication A form of communication that involves gestures and body language, often used by non- or pre-speaking autistic children.

Reasonable adjustments Adjustments that an organisation (school or setting) or service provider should make to reduce disadvantage for disabled people.

Frame The way a specific subject or idea is conceptualised and explained, which may or may not include bias and opinion.

Stigma Negative and unfair belief associated with a person, set of people or situation.

Bias Unreasonable and unfair judgement of a person or group.

Ideology A set of cultural ideas and beliefs on which a society bases its structures, systems, policies and processes.

Deficit-based model Focuses on the needs or weaknesses within a person or group of people, such that that group comes to be seen as having inherent problems. This model fails to consider the challenges such groups experience.

Ableism A form of discrimination. It is characterised by the belief that individuals with physical, mental, or developmental atypicality need to be fixed.[5]

Masking 'A psychological safety mechanism made up of complex layers of physical, emotional and social actions which an autistic person is driven to use to self-protect and project an acceptable version of who they are.'[6]

5   R. Casteneda and M. Peters, "Ableism," In: M. Adams, W. J. Blumenfeld, R. Castaneda, H. W. Hackman, M. Peters and X. Zuniga, Eds., Reading for Diversity and Social Justice: An Anthology on Racism, Antisemitism, Sexism, Heterosexism, Ableism, and Classism, Routledge, New York, 2000, pp. 310-325.

6   The Autistic Advocate. (n.d.). Autistic Masking resources from Kieran Rose, The Autistic Advocate. [online] Available at: https:// theautisticadvocate.com/autistic-masking/.

PART ONE:

WHERE WE ARE AND HOW WE GOT HERE

I want to open a discussion about the ways we, as a society, currently frame and understand autism. Until recently, sensory experiences have not featured as an important part of the autistic story. The focus has been on changing behaviours identified as unexpected and unusual. Therefore, in this initial part, I will touch only briefly on the sensory aspects of autistic profiles. Through deconstructing the way we currently view autism, I will attempt to show how assumptions made about autistic traits often lead to inappropriate supports, environments and expectations.

Where we are now

A little girl aged five sits in a waiting room; the room has white walls and a shiny, plain white floor. The girl has ignored all the little chairs around her and instead sits on the cold floor surrounded by toys. For the last fifteen minutes, she has been playing with a toy of large, brightly coloured wooden beads threaded onto a thick green wire. As she pushes the beads across the wire, she smiles and speaks to herself in sounds and words that few would understand except her parents. This little girl's name is Joannie. Joannie looks up at her parents as they whisper to one another in hushed tones; she studies them from across the room with wide eyes. Joannie's parents stop whispering when they notice her looking over; she seems perplexed or concerned, and her mum and dad automatically smile at their daughter reassuringly. Joannie seems to relax slightly and returns to spinning and pushing the large beads from one side of the wire to the other, whispering as she plays.

Joannie's mum watches her daughter and holds her breath; she has a tight feeling in her chest and hates that they are all sitting in this clinical, cold white room waiting for an appointment she has been dreading for weeks. Thoughts had run through her mind of how Joannie would cope, what the doctor might be like and what they might be told during the appointment. Joannie's mum is broken out of her thoughts when Joannie suddenly spins a bead all the way across the wire and giggles gleefully, flapping her hands quickly and tensing her little body with excitement. 'How could anyone think my daughter is broken or wrong?' Joannie's mum thinks to herself. 'She is glorious!'

They are called into their appointment. Joannie's mum tenses once more. She is tense because she is too used to being told by everyone how her daughter is struggling. At Joannie's nursery, they had daily reports of Joannie's unwillingness to play with others. Each morning, Joannie cried as she was pulled from her mother's arms, reaching out with scared eyes as they carried her into the room. In reception, things improved, but they still heard how Joannie tried to escape and refused to play with other children. Her parents considered homeschooling her but were told by others around them that she would be better off with other children her own age. When Joannie was three, discussions had begun about her lack of speech and progress, and it was agreed that she should be assessed for her social communication needs.

The appointment is short. The paediatrician listens to Joannie's parents talk about their daughter; she smiles kindly. She observes Joannie and diagnoses what they had all thought: Joannie is autistic. A mixture of trepidation and relief washes over her parents. Joannie's dad feels this will be the beginning of his daughter getting the support she needs and asks about the next steps. He is told of long waiting lists and of support taking years to access. They are given information leaflets and a list of charities that support autistic children. Emotionally drained and deflated, Joannie's dad picks her up; she reaches out and traces her finger

3

across his face with her soft little fingers. Her dad softly kisses her on her forehead, making her eyes crinkle and sparkle. A wordless conversation like so many before, hard to explain but unequivocally there.

The deficit-based model

These non-spoken moments of communication are not logged anywhere in the description of autism or even discussed in relation to autism. Yet it will be a story familiar to parents of autistic children everywhere. Young autistic children often find ways of communicating that break the mould, such as leading people towards an item they want, crying to show their distress, touching foreheads to show affection or flapping with delight. These unspoken communication traits vary from child to child and from family to family, but autistic communication is an important marker of internal processes that are often overlooked in the diagnosis process. Instead, parents are confronted with a list of traits that mark all the ways their autistic child is 'failing'. The current method of identifying autistic children is based on a medicalised model of behavioural profiling, where a professional (such as a paediatrician or diagnostician) observes a child who has been flagged as falling behind. The professional logs the child's traits against the behaviours listed in diagnostic manuals. If the child scores highly enough (exhibits enough traits), they are diagnosed as autistic.

The current diagnostic criteria in the DSM5[7] lists behaviours such as:[8]

- Persistent social communication deficits include gestures, body language and abnormal eye contact.
- Deficits in using social communication, such as greetings and social sharing.
- Impairments in changing the style of communication to suit other people and contexts (such as moving from the playground to the classroom).
- Difficulties following rules for conversation, such as turn-taking and rephrasing.
- Difficulties understanding what is not explicitly stated (e.g., making inferences).
- Deficits in developing and maintaining relationships and difficulties with imaginative play.
- Insistence on sameness, inflexible routines, ritualised patterns of behaviour, difficulties with minor changes, transitions and disordered rigid thinking patterns.
- Stereotyped and repetitive movements and speech, including lining things up, echopraxia (motor repetition) and echolalia (verbal repetition).

---

7   American Psychiatric Association (2013). Diagnostic and Statistical Manual of Mental Disorders. 5th ed. American Psychiatric Publishing.

8   Centers for Disease Control and Prevention (2016). Autism Spectrum Disorder Diagnostic Criteria. [online] Centers for Disease Control and Prevention. Available at: https://www.cdc.gov/ncbddd/autism/hcp-dsm.html.

- Abnormal restricted and intense interests and an unusual attachment to objects.
- Hyper- or hypo-reactivity to sensory input or unusual interests in sensory aspects of the environment.

These traits are based on a deficit-based model where unusual behaviours are marked out as problematic. It is distressing to be told that your child is lacking in all these areas, and this is often reinforced through conversations with nurseries and schools (just as it was for Joannie's parents). Being given the above diagnosis and a handful of leaflets leaves many parents wondering where to turn. It is my opinion (and the opinion of many autistic adults, advocates and allies) that the diagnosis process and the above descriptions of autistic traits are deeply flawed. A diagnosis based on profiling autistic traits through observation can only tell a story of what can be *seen*. Even the most recent addition of sensory reactivity only labels *observable* responses. Observable traits are surface markers of the rich internal world that autistic children experience. Joannie's traits of looking at her parents with feeling in her eyes, her gleeful flapping hands and her non-spoken communication are all marked out as deficits, difficulties and restrictions in the above diagnosis. But what if the opposite were true? What if Joannie's traits were considered meaningful?

As an early years teacher and parent, I have personally observed any number of baffling traits displayed by both non-autistic and autistic children. These traits can seem nonsensical to the observer but are almost always very meaningful to the children. For example, repetition can be extremely meaningful, and many young children's play can include such traits. It is well known that most children go through a stage of schematic play where babies, toddlers and young children are involved in repeated actions or behaviours as they explore their environment. In non-autistic children, repetition is not seen as abnormal or deficit-based. This type of play is described as appropriate play that aids development. But when autistic children use repetition (often with more intensity than their non-autistic peers or at an age when the trait is unexpected), little mention is made of the meaningful nature of these traits. The current diagnosis leads some parents to think their child embodies all the words in the diagnosis and that they are in some way broken and in need of fixing. Often, the end goal for parents and professionals becomes minimising behaviours deemed to be autistic traits. Many autistic children are steered towards the expected, such as sustaining eye contact and joining in group play, with a focus on helping the autistic child to act more like a non-autistic child.

How have we moved so far from seeing autistic traits as meaningful and useful? How has autistic communication and socialising become marked out as a problem that needs fixing? Much of this has happened because our understanding of autism has developed through the handing down of 'knowledge' from generation to generation. Knowledge passed down this way, especially based on scientific research, is not often questioned. It is taken as fact. Systems, structures, policies and social rules grow around this knowledge (often called 'socially constructed knowledge').

By following the journey of how autism has been socially constructed, it is possible to see how old-fashioned and outdated ideas feed into modern-day diagnoses and therapies. Although socially constructed ideas do change and develop as new scientific research becomes available, in the case of autism, these changes have been slow to materialise. Many of the descriptions of autistic traits listed in the autism diagnosis are over one hundred years old.

How did we get here?

To understand how we got here, we need to go back to the 1850s and a lady called Pauline Bleuler.[9] Pauline was born in Switzerland in 1852 and had a brother named Eugene, who was five years younger than her. Both Eugene and Pauline experienced synaesthesia (described as the blending of sensory information). Specifically, they had chromesthesia, sound-to-colour synaesthesia, where a person might view musical notes as different colours. This trait is often associated with advanced musical abilities. Pauline was indeed a talented musician and worked as a piano

---

9   Brückner, Burkhart. (2015). Biographical entry: Anna Pauline Bleuler (1852-1926).

teacher for many years. She also had some sort of synaesthesia around vowels and words. This latter type of synaesthesia presents in many ways; for example, 'colour to letter' synaesthesia is a phenomenon where different letters are visualised as different colours. It is important to note that Eugene's firsthand experience of chromesthesia and his observations of his sister gave him an inside-out understanding of how sensory profiles can differ between people. His knowledge of a rich sensory inner world was partly from his own lived experience.

Around 1882, when Pauline was in her thirties, she experienced an extreme mental health crisis and was placed in an asylum (as was the practice at the time). Pauline's crisis was described as 'catatonic mutism', which included speech difficulties, freezing episodes and mobility issues. While in the asylum, Pauline refused to eat and showed signs of distress. She also displayed behaviours that others found challenging, including instances of self-harm, biting and a tendency to throw things. Force and restraint were used to 'deal' with Pauline's behaviours. Institutionalisation and restraint were commonplace at this time: many people whose behaviour fell significantly outside of what was expected were removed from their families and frequently treated appallingly. It is safe to assume that many asylum patients were autistic. Indeed, Pauline Bleuler presented with many traits associated with the modern-day diagnosis of regressive autism (where communication and motor skills can be lost over time).[10]

Pauline's experiences seem to have had a profound effect on Eugene. He studied to become a psychologist and cared for his sister following the death of his parents in 1889. Eugene opposed using force, possibly due to its adverse effects on his sister. Instead, he cared for her at his clinic and then at home, believing that repetitive gentle suggestions and demonstrations could create better outcomes than force. He spent hours gently communicating with Pauline, successfully creating a shared understanding.

In his work as a psychologist, Eugene studied matters of the mind and coined the term schizophrenia (which he stated was a splitting of the mind). He used his experiences with his sister and other patients to develop four primary symptoms, and it was here that the term autism was first used. The etymology of this word came from 'auto', meaning *self,* and 'ism', meaning *a state or condition.* He grouped autistic behaviours with other behaviours he had observed in his patients under the diagnosis of schizophrenia. These included abnormal associations, autistic behaviour and thinking, abnormal affect and ambivalence.

Eugene described autistic behaviour and thinking as an infantile wish to escape difficult realities through revelling in fantasies and hallucinations. He stated that

10   Evans, B. (2013). How autism became autism. History of the Human Sciences, [online] 26(3), pp.3–31. Available at: https://www. ncbi.nlm.nih.gov/pmc/articles/PMC3757918/.

the autistic 'inner life' and fantasies were not accessible to observers. Eugene believed these traits could become progressively more noticeable in some patients, culminating in the presentation of schizophrenic dementia, which Eugene described as a loss of skills. In his view, each person's outcome (whether traits would become more or less pronounced) depended on their capacity to adapt and also on their environmental circumstances. Eugene continued his narrative that people who presented with 'catatonia', like his sister, could be influenced through gentle suggestions.

I cannot help but think that if we had followed the example of Eugene Bleuler's support for his sister, autistic people might have been given more time to develop along their own timeline and possibly have experienced less stigma. Bleuler was a product of his time and had many ableist and unsavoury ideas about dealing with unexpected traits. But he also seemed to have an empathetic approach in other areas, advocating to normalise hereditary sensory experiences. It is possible that Eugene's emotional connection with his sister and his own sensory experiences of synaesthesia may have underpinned his advocacy for gentle support.

During the 1920s, many psychologists, psychoanalysts and psychiatrists in England used the term *autism* in line with Eugene's ideas of a rich inner world. Jean Piaget, arguably one of the most important developmental psychologists of the twentieth century, tied autism in with his theories on how children construct their understanding of the world through language[11]. Piaget considered young children to be in an egocentric state (thinking only of themselves) until their spoken language developed sufficiently that they could move into understanding the thoughts and ideas of others. He suggested that autistic children did not progress past the initial stages of this process and became stuck in something he termed 'magical imagination', where concrete concepts had not yet been embedded. This narrative was much more concerned with the inner world of autistic children. Unfortunately, these ideas were about to be relegated to the history books with regard to autism. Although Piaget's ideas are still taught in teacher training today and are used to conceptualise how children learn, neither his nor Bleuler's ideas continued to inform the autistic narrative.

Instead, a new breed of psychologists became instrumental in shaping the way autism was framed; these psychologists rejected introspective methods, which were concerned with inner emotions and feelings, and instead sought to understand traits only by measuring observable behaviours and events. In the 1940s, B.F. Skinner, an American psychologist, introduced a theory of learning called operant conditioning[12], stating that learning and behaviour

11   Evans, B. (2013). How autism became autism. History of the Human Sciences, [online] 26(3), pp.3–31. Available at: https://www.ncbi.nlm.nih.gov/pmc/articles/PMC3757918/.

12   Cherry, K. (2020). B. F. Skinner Biography. [online] Verywell Mind. Available at: https://www.verywellmind.com/b-f-skinner-biography-1904-1990-2795543.

could be impacted through positive and negative reinforcement. This was based on animal behaviours but was soon to be used on humans through a model called radical behaviourism.

Around the same time, autism was also being completely reconceptualised through this behaviourist model. This would flip Eugene Bleuler's original idea that autistic people had rich inner worlds and vivid imaginations, and state the complete opposite, that autistic people were devoid of imagination. These psychologists and psychiatrists have been instrumental in constructing the autistic narrative still used today. At this point, Bleuler's advocacy for gentle and patient instruction was lost entirely.

The myth of normal and behaviourist approaches

Leo Kanner[13] was one such psychiatrist. In 1943, Kanner was working at John Hopkins University Hospital in Baltimore when he wrote a paper about children who diverged considerably from their peers and showed 'fascinating peculiarities'. He asserted that these children showed little interest in the social world and instead focused on objects in their surroundings,

---

13   Cohmer, S. (2014). Early Infantile Autism and the Refrigerator Mother Theory (1943-1970) | The Embryo Project Encyclopedia. [online] Asu.edu. Available at: https://embryo.asu.edu/pages/ear ly-infantile-autism-and-refrigerator-mother-theory-1943-1970.

displaying a desire for aloneness. He called this 'condition' early infantile autism. Soon after, in his 1944 paper, Hans Asperger, an Austrian psychiatrist, wrote about another group of children who presented with fleeting eye contact, a lack of imaginative play, impaired sensory and spatial awareness, and behavioural issues. The behaviours identified by Kanner and Asperger may seem very similar to the traits of autism, which are still used today, and that is because they *are* similar. Despite significant advancements in our scientific comprehension of the brain and internal processes in recent years, these insights have yet to fully impact the autism diagnostic criteria, which are still based on identifying observable behaviours.

Both Kanner and Asperger felt these behaviours were so 'abnormal' that the children they identified needed to be treated with medical and psychological interventions, which were often highly damaging to the autistic people they were inflicted upon. This included many awful therapies I will not go into, but if you wish to look these up, you will find some quite odious practices. The main approach that both men advocated for was the behaviourist approach. In the case of autistic children, it was thought that a regime of punishment for unexpected behaviours and rewards for expected behaviours would condition these children to use more acceptable behaviours. Although this process did change behaviours, it is known to have been highly distressing and traumatising for the autistic participants.

Behaviourist approaches are still implemented with

many autistic children through current therapies. Although these have been re-packaged to offer positive reinforcement when autistic children display 'expected' behaviours, while leaving out the punishment for 'unexpected' behaviours, the issue with such practices is that behaviourist therapies remove children's autonomy. Any learning the child makes is not based on that child's intrinsic drive; instead, the instructor holds all the power over what the child 'should' learn and do.

For example, if a child attempts to escape a busy nursery room filled with children and noise, the approach of a behaviourist practitioner might be to conclude that the child's avoidant behaviour needs to be rectified. They might offer reinforcement by allowing the child access to their favourite toy when they agree to stay in the room. But what if the underlying cause for trying to leave was how loud and busy the classroom felt to them? Now, the child is sitting quietly in the room with their toy, but they are still experiencing the noise and may feel overwhelmed by the busyness. This interaction has only taught them to suppress their distress and to pretend they are fine in moments of overwhelm. They may still feel tense stress, almost like a coiled spring. When that child goes out to play in a bustling playground, they are much more likely to be tipped into behaviour that others may deem challenging. That is because the behaviourist practitioner has overridden their expression of autonomy over what their body needs.

This persistent idea that autistic children are broken is pervasive: it still runs through every part of how we view autism today. Prominent researchers who have built the autism narrative over the last sixty years have all created theories by working from this deficit-based model. These include the concept of the 'triad of impairments', which outlines deficits in various areas for autistic individuals, encompassing social and emotional interaction, social communication, language, imagination, and flexibility of thought. Another theory is that of Weak Central Coherence, later referred to as simply Central Coherence[14], which highlights the limited capacity of autistic individuals to perceive context or 'see the bigger picture'. A further idea is that of a deficit in 'theory of mind',[15] [16] wherein autistic individuals are theorised to struggle to infer the thoughts and feelings of others and can experience challenges in empathising. Lastly, the 'executive (dys)function'[17] model portrays deficits in cognitive functions like planning, maintaining focus, remembering instructions, and effectively managing multiple tasks.

All these theories assume incompetence on the part of the autistic individual, and all continue to feed into

14   Frith, U. (1989). Explaining the enigma. [online] Blackwell. Available at: https://www.wiley.com/en-us/Autism%3A+Explain ing+the+Enigma%2C+2nd+Edition-p-9780631229018.

15   Baron-Cohen, S., Leslie, A.M. and Frith, U. (1985). Does the Autistic Child Have a 'Theory of Mind'? Cognition, 21(1), pp.37–46. doi:https://doi.org/10.1016/0010-0277(85)90022-8.

16   Pennington, B.F. (1997). Dimensions of executive functions in normal and abnormal development.

17   Russell, J. (1997). Autism as an executive disorder. Oxford: Oxford University Press

the design of places and practices that support autistic children (such as therapies, policies, nurseries and schools). They offer a list of expected traits which autistic children are not attaining. There is no discussion in any of these research papers about what autistic children may be learning instead of the expected. Nothing delves into how they access the sensory world and how their autistic communication, socialisation, learning profiles, and developmental trajectories might differ from their non-autistic peers.

We should understand that many people who fed into the autism narrative throughout history often did so with altruistic intentions. However, research framed through the deficit-based model has caused trauma to the autistic community, and until very recently, this has been the *only* type of research available. It can be difficult to see how changing a research narrative could positively impact autistic children themselves. The current narrative creates unseen bias that impacts autistic people's everyday lives. It frames autistic children as broken and in need of fixing instead of considering the incompatible and inhospitable environments and social settings in which they are meant to thrive.

Who gets to decide?

Research can often feel detached and distant from the lives we live. How could our day-to-day lives be influenced by someone sitting in a lab testing where a child's gaze is focused or whether a child can read another person's emotions? Having now studied in the field of autism, it is apparent to me that research touches and shapes so much of the lives we experience. For hundreds of years, research has been conducted by the people who hold the most power in each country; in the UK, that has been mostly non-disabled, white men. This means their ideas of what to research, who to research, and how to research, and their opinions and unconscious biases have greatly influenced our everyday lives. The consequences of research bias are hidden in plain sight in our daily practices, and it can be overwhelming when you begin to notice the degree of influence powerful players in society have over us.

The best way to uncover this unseen influence is to describe how such influences, such as hierarchies, were established in human history. This means going back to long before governments, capitalism, nurseries, and schools even existed. Thousands of years ago, humans lived as nomadic hunter-gatherers in small groups. There was no wider society, hence no societal rules. Life was about surviving day by day. While there is evidence of a rudimentary hierarchy (rooted in physical dominance) during this period, the introduction of weaponry shifted such dominance to a more level playing field. Consequently, it is believed that these groups organised themselves to hunt cooperatively.

Anthropologists believe humans began to settle into communities around twelve thousand to fourteen thousand years ago. Such communities would change the course of human lives. So began the formation of societies and socially constructed narratives and expectations. It is thought that humans organised themselves into larger groups to farm crops and animals. Around this time, more organised hierarchical systems and structures began, where some people within communities held more power. The masterminds of agricultural processes often became leaders and amassed resources and land, and passed these on to future generations. Alongside this, the value of each person (and each family) in the community became more tied to their ability to contribute to the advancement of that community. Unseen influences of judgement and social expectation grew around work, religion, families, power and belongings.

These structures, systems and ideologies were constructed through social interactions and conversations where judgement about a person's ability fed into stigma and inequality.[18] People who had been useful hunter-gatherers were required to adapt and learn new skills. Those deemed to lack the expected skills needed for agriculture were likely labelled as 'less' – less useful and less skilled. This also meant people's ideas about themselves (their self-perception) became more tied to how much they could conform to develop expected skills and how others in the community judged them.

---

18   Perret, C., Hart, E. and Powers, S.T. (2020). From disorganized equality to efficient hierarchy: how group size drives the evolution of hierarchy in human societies. Proceedings of the Royal Society B: Biological Sciences, 287(1928), p.20200693. doi:https://doi.org/10.1098/rspb.2020.0693.

It is hard to understand why humans fell so easily into following the rules of powerful people within hierarchies. It seems strange that anyone would accept the position of being a follower and adhere to the expectations of others whom they deem more powerful because of their status. But this often happens because people believe they have no choice. Humans have navigated a path, evolving from nomadic hunter-gatherers who made decisions primarily for their personal survival and well-being to our contemporary era where, in certain respects, we find ourselves with diminished autonomy over our own lives. In the UK, we may feel we have complete autonomy over our lives and our children's lives. But do we? We still adhere to largely hidden socially constructed rules, and nowhere is that more apparent than in the way children's behaviours and traits are managed and moulded throughout their lives to fit a socially constructed narrative based on an 'expected' developmental pathway.

Milestones and expectations

In many ways, our modern-day construction of how human children 'should' be is tightly managed. There are certain expectations from birth based on the age when children *should* start walking, potty training, talking and even pointing. There is an expected pathway of development, and in England and Wales this is enshrined in documents such as:

- Birth to 5 Matters (non-statutory guidance for the Early Years Foundation Stage)[19]
- The Early Years Foundation Stage (EYFS)[20]
- The National Curriculum[21]

These documents list expected developmental targets that babies and children 'should' hit. Our whole system of monitoring babies, toddlers and children is based on the idea that human babies are born with similar brains, bodies and sensory systems. Therefore, they will hit certain milestones and access similar learned concepts at a similar age. An autistic baby is born with a brain and a sensory system that is not 'standardised' and does not fit this 'expected' developmental pathway. Often, parents of autistic babies are left confused and worried because their experience of being a new parent is not represented in any baby book. The advice many professionals give often does not work for their baby in one regard or another. The baby may be labelled as a poor sleeper, an excessive crier, a fussy eater or a baby

---

19   Early Education (2021). Birth to 5 Matters: Non-statutory guidance for the Early Years Foundation Stage www.birthto5matters.org.uk From the Early Years Coalition. [online] Available at: https://birthto5matters.org.uk/wp-content/uploads/2021/04/Birth to5Matters-download.pdf.

20   Department for Education (2021). Early years foundation stage statutory framework (EYFS). [online] GOV.UK. Available at: https://www.gov.uk/government/publications/early-years-foundation-stage-framework--2.

21   Department for Education (2013). National Curriculum. [online] GOV.UK. Available at: https://www.gov.uk/government/collections/national-curriculum.

with attachment issues. Whatever the label, autistic development in babies is often labelled as unfavourable. Parents may be given the impression that their baby is not interacting as a proper human baby should.

These parents often feel pressure to help their children 'catch up' and can choose from various therapies that assist with this goal. Many take their children to potty training classes, sleep workshops and baby weaning training, to name but a few. But these expectations and targets are often based on the 'average child'. In child development, hitting these averages is tied to specific ages. This means all children are tasked with hitting at least the 50th percentile in expected skills at specific ages. This is a nonsensical system; every population will have outliers: children who hit milestones earlier, those who hit milestones later and those who were never going to hit those expected milestones at all. By definition, half of all kids will not hit milestones 'on time'.

Children who do not reach 'expected' milestones by a specific age are marked out as being behind, and those who hit them early are viewed as advanced. But life is not a race, and it is not the natural order that *all* children should hit these milestones at the same age. Children who are developing divergent skills will likely not hit many 'expected' milestones on time. So why are children compared and judged so rigidly against each other when it comes to expected milestones? These milestones assist with the smooth running of society, including the idea that children should move into nursery and school settings at a given age. Therefore, there is pressure on parents to get children 'school ready'.

Conformity goes hand in hand with early years and school settings. Having a room of thirty children with only a few staff members means that these settings need children to follow rules to keep everything running smoothly. Parents are usually asked to ensure their child is potty trained by the age of four at the latest, as it is not always feasible for teachers and assistants to change children's nappies during school. Stigma can follow those who cannot help their child to reach these targets on time.

This is also the case when a child struggles to follow behaviour expectations in a setting. A child who becomes distressed in a conventional setting may need to leave the setting for some time to regulate. This need or requirement might not be easily accommodated due to staffing levels. Behaviour concerns are instead often reported to the parents, placing the responsibility on parents to help their children conform to behaviour expectations. For autistic children who may develop skills in different ways and at different times to their peers, this can be an anxiety-inducing time for parents and children alike.

Things can become even more complex when autistic children move on to primary school. These settings of at least thirty children in each class are busy, noisy places with huge amounts of sensory input both in classrooms and in playgrounds. There is minimal opportunity for downtime when children can unplug from environmental intrusions. The early-years philosophy of following a child's interests to encourage them to be life-long learners stops abruptly from Year 1 in England and Wales (and probably in many other countries). Instead, primary schools encourage even more conformity with more sitting at desks and listening to teachers. Knowledgeable teachers aim to teach children in the most creative ways possible, incorporating differentiated learning and kinaesthetic elements. Still, the restrictions of the National Curriculum mean that teachers are limited in what and how they can teach.

Are schools truly inclusive for all children?

There is a persistent belief that modern schools are organised to create the optimal environment for all children to learn. For thousands of years before schools existed, humans amassed vast amounts of knowledge by following their intrinsic interests. But schools are not organised around areas of interest. Instead, they are organised by age and by subject. In the UK, the government has influence over what children are expected to learn and by what age through a variety of policies. Teachers are then tasked with teaching and testing children on set age-related expectations. The children who find this style of learning and testing at odds with their learning profile might then be framed as lacking the expected skills for their age. Children's school reports then pass this information to parents, and often, they seek advice on how to help their child catch up.

It is crucial to highlight that if schools were designed to cater to diverse learning profiles, including those where children reach certain academic milestones at different times, it could help mitigate the stigma associated with autistic children appearing to 'fall behind' their peers. For many autistic children, this process of attempting to fit into a schooling system built around expected development can be anxiety-inducing. If children's mental health is affected when these systems and structures do not serve them, they are not allowed to rest and recover; instead, governments can fine and prosecute parents for missed school days. So, is it the case that schools are optimal learning environments for *all* children?

Many autistic children must contend with a daily barrage of sensory stimuli. The journey to school can be an exhausting experience in itself, filled with car noises, plane noise, busy streets and even the wind whistling or the sun shining brightly. In mainstream schools, sensory input can be intensified by the presence of large groups of children generating noise. The majority of children may be happy in such environments, but for children who experience the sensory world differently from the majority, such environments may not be optimal. Couple this with the fact that current learning and testing systems may not suit their learning profiles, and this means many children struggle to thrive at school. When parents pull their children out of these settings and homeschool their children, they are often harshly judged for rejecting an 'expected' pathway. But many parents do this to avoid further traumatising their children. This is not to say that *all* schools traumatise *all* autistic children, but that it is harder to meet autistic requirements in the current schooling system.

There are multiple ways that neurosensory divergent children experience trauma in such settings. Many of the systems, structures and policies we currently have are based on research around what is best for the majority of children. This neglects to consider the detrimental effect that the system might have on minority groups. Measuring autistic children against non-autistic children is problematic in many ways, due to their different profiles. So why is society obsessed with this system? Many of the measures applied to children's development were initially put in place for altruistic reasons. These measures aimed to identify potential medical conditions for early intervention, provide support for vulnerable children, and guarantee a comprehensive education for all. Somewhere along this journey, society has lost sight of diversity as a natural part of human development; instead, these systems seek to bring all children in line with one another.

When policymakers fail to validate autistic development and still view autism as either a behavioural or cognitive disorder, they may be less inclined to allocate funding to autistic causes. Setting up schools that meet autistic requirements or changing the current schooling system would be a costly business. Many parents of autistic children know their child requires a different type of education, but there are very few options. Special school places are extremely limited and often fail to cater for all autistic children.

I believe that if neurosensory divergent profiles (including spiky learning profiles) were better understood, more parents could advocate for their autistic child's needs. This fight to have schools that are equitable for those with sensory divergence is the same fight that parents of deaf and blind children face. Autistic children need an education system that is built around their learning and sensory profiles. Being in the minority does not make children less deserving of a robust and tailored education.

Seeing beyond our system

During my teacher training, diversity was touched upon, but the idea of socially constructed systems, structures and the social models which we operate within were not discussed. This is because this training course was not attempting to shift a narrative or change the way society thinks. My teaching qualification was designed to reinforce current ideas about how children learn. It was not until I enrolled on an autism masters course that I really got to grips with the concept of social constructs; these teachings opened my eyes to the way natural human divergence is often stigmatised when the 'ways of being' of the majority are favoured.

Research often feeds into theories that promote a one-size-fits-all approach to settings and education. For example, current ideologies around unstructured times at school (e.g. playtimes, lunchtimes) are based on the idea that children need time at school when they are not in a 'taught' environment so they can relax. Often, children form social groups in playgrounds; they might engage in play based on talking or around a sport. The barriers many autistic children face during unstructured times are not always fully understood. Autistic children may not play or communicate in the same way as their non-autistic peers. They may have motor barriers to joining in with sports. They may feel overwhelmed by the busyness of the playground and yet need the regulating movement of running and playing. Although many schools implement supports, such as lunchtime clubs and quiet times in libraries, this is usually set up by individual schools. There is no policy that details the effects sensory and communication divergence can have on some children. This narrative gap is likely due to the lack of autistic voices in educational research.

This one-size-fits-all approach also influences policies that govern teaching and learning. For example, the current system of teaching reading (in most UK mainstream schools) is based on the idea that *all* children can learn to read effectively through systematic synthetic phonics (matching sounds to letters and groups of letters). From the many cohorts of children I have worked with, I can tell you this simply isn't true. Many autistic children read via whole sight word reading (where they remember whole words). Some struggle to remember written words and instead need pictures to help them with their reading acquisition. Other children (such as dyslexic children) need a completely different system altogether. Early testing of phonics meant that if a child did not learn via this style of teaching and learning, they were marked out as a struggling reader. It is important to point out that if these children were taught in an optimal way for their learning profile, they may not struggle at all.

Without the input of autistic and neurodivergent voices, these children's experiences of playtime and class time may not be explicitly apparent. To create a fairer society, research and policy decision-makers should always include a cross-section of voices from different minority groups, including autistic groups. Those who are being researched deserve a place at the head table.

As a teacher, it was soul-destroying to have to teach via systems and structures that benefitted the majority but acted as a barrier to learning for so many children in my classroom. I was given ever more prescriptive manuals that told me how to teach and removed my autonomy and creativity in teaching how different children *needed* me to teach them. Even if there had been time to implement alternative learning systems for the minority (which there was not), teachers were not 'supposed' to offer a different style of learning. While differentiation was encouraged, where children were given learning materials appropriate for their academic level, this still did not allow for different teaching ideologies to be implemented. For example, I could not teach whole-word spelling alongside synthetic phonics. I was expected to stick to the National Curriculum and follow the set teaching programmes in favour at the time.

In England, the Education Secretary and the Education Department are tasked with deciding which educational theories should influence policy: our political parties are made up of mostly non-disabled, white men. The Education Department does bring in groups and panels to advise them on policy, but often, they use organisations that support autistic children, as opposed to getting lived experiences from the groups themselves. While the Education Department is made up of civil servants, many of whom have had direct teaching experience, it is ultimately the people in charge who make the final call on what will be implemented.

I must clarify: I have nothing against England's majority demographic – non-disabled, white men – my father is one, and I am married to one! But they are *not* best placed to understand my experience of the world as a neurodivergent woman who is part of multiple marginalised groups, and I would suggest they are not best placed to understand educational best practice for autistic children. If the people who decide on educational policy have not experienced ableism, racism, sexism or any other kind of marginalisation, and if these people have been in the majority and been mostly served by the majority systems and structures, then are they best placed to decide how *all* children learn effectively?

In this way, bias can impact the kind of research that is carried out and the choices made about which research to follow. Research that is in favour under one political party will be completely different from research in favour under another political party. This means that the ideology (ideas and ideals) that influences policies (such as the national curriculum) changes completely when a new party takes over. This means teachers' working practices change, too, and the way children are taught changes.

In educational research, some research papers state that children learn best when sitting and listening to input from a knowledgeable teacher, where the teacher imparts information and children are rewarded for retaining this information, thus reinforcing the learning (this is a behaviourist stance). However, other researchers have 'proved' that children learn best when learning in a self-directed manner, where they have access to different learning opportunities in their environment and where they are guided by the teacher, who is seen as a knowledgeable facilitator to the child's natural exploratory process (this is a child-centred approach). This means that the ruling political party can pick and choose whatever research serves their own ideology and implement policies that impact teachers, parents, children, and society as a whole.

Many people who thrive in our current schooling and working environments do so because it was designed around their experiences of the world. It is extremely important to be aware of who has designed the world we exist in because it helps to explain why life can be such a struggle for those who experience the world differently from the majority. It is not because they are in some way lacking as human beings but because their style of learning, working and thriving looks different from the way the majority learn, work and thrive. In the case of autistic children, I hope to show how Neurosensory Divergent profiles necessitate the development of new best practice for supporting that divergence. Expecting autistic children to thrive in environments and belief systems that actively work to prove they are lacking or broken is highly problematic.

Viewing autism from the inside

The study of autism has conventionally fallen under the social sciences, which is concerned with studying societies and the relationships among individuals within those societies. The social science researchers who have been most instrumental in describing and categorising autism have been researchers in the field of psychology. Psychology has gone through something of a crisis recently, where the credibility of psychological research has been called into question. Studies are thought to be scientifically sound when the experiments conducted by researchers can be repeated to produce the same results. However, researching human beings in the same way as one conducts a chemistry experiment will always run into problems. Human beings are messy:

we do not fit easily into groupings, because of our varied experiences, beliefs, bodies, brains and so on. That makes the psychological study of homogenous groups (people who are alike in some way) very difficult.

As I've explained, the societal norms we encounter from birth shape our perception of the world and the people in it. This exposure can lead to the development of biases, including racism and gender bias. Often, these biases manifest as unconscious biases, where individuals may not be fully aware of their held views, as they have become deeply ingrained. Research (especially research around human development) can be highly subjective – that is, it is affected by the individual's personal beliefs and understanding of the world. One such bias that impacts autistic people is the assumption that people who are unable to speak are less cognitively able (this type of thinking is ableist as it assumes incompetence). This assumption has meant that historically, non-speaking autistic people were often taught only basic skills. Although it may be the case that some autistic children have learning difficulties, many autistic children have proved such assumptions to be incorrect. Clearly, this assumption may be doing lots of autistic people a disservice.

Traditional autism research often attempts to group autistic children as experiencing the world in the same way. As with the children in my classroom, a 'one-size-fits-all' approach to studying cohorts of children does not often yield results that lead to best practice. Each autistic child has a story about how they experience the world. This does not have to be a spoken story; it can also be told in activities, traits and interactions. Jim Sinclair, an autistic advocate, penned an article in 1993 entitled 'Don't Mourn for Us'[22]. In it, he explains that engaging with autistic children takes effort on the part of others to relate to autistic languages and 'ways of being', stating that autistic traits are often purposeful and meaningful. This framing is a far cry from traditional autism research, where autistic children are often deemed unable to explain competently or show why they behave in a certain way. Researchers need to step away from the idea that autistic children must cease their behaviours in favour of non-autistic behaviours and instead look to what autistic autonomy might lead to, where autistic children drive the narrative around their favoured environments and types of interactions.

The main problem with non-autistic people diagnosing and framing autistic behaviours is that they cannot see autism from the inside. They can only base their understanding of autistic behaviours on their own experiences, which are likely to differ significantly from autistic experiences. For example, autistic children and adults often describe their sensory experiences of the world in ways that many non-autistic people have never experienced. Donna Williams[23], an autistic author, said in

---

22 Sinclair, J. (2012). DON'T MOURN FOR US. [online] 1(1). Available at: https://philosophy.ucsc.edu/SinclairDontMournForUs. pdf.

23 Williams, D. (1999). Nobody Nowhere: the remarkable autobi-ography of an autistic girl. London: Jessica Kingsley.

her book *Nobody Nowhere* that her sensory experiences could sometimes feel beautiful and hypnotic, and she would feel spellbound by colour and sensations. In contrast, she found voices to be an intrusion that would break into her joy.

Similarly, Anand Prahlad[24], a black author who identifies as Aspergers[25]*, says he often does not hear words as most people do. Instead, he sees words in his mind, listens to their colours and smells their scent. He explains that although he uses the same words as other people, he often feels like he is speaking a different language. Inside-out accounts like this offer a new perspective. Autistic people who speak from their own experiences seem to hit roadblocks at every turn when attempting to move the narrative forward. Traditional researchers are still churning out papers that list problematic autistic behaviours: their inability to move on from this narrative of deficit, delay, and disorder is frustrating. You could almost call it restricted thinking.

Research and scientific discoveries are fallible – mistakes can be made. Science includes discoveries believed to be true today and past truths that have subsequently been disproved. The Greeks, for example, believed in Humourism; this ancient medical theory

---

24   Anand Prahlad (2017). The secret life of a Black Aspie: a memoir. Fairbanks, Ak: University of Alaska Press.

25   *This is a term which is no longer used diagnostically and is seen by many as controversial due to Asperger's connection to the Nazis, but it is still used by some autistic people who feel connected to this identity

posited that the human body is composed of four primary humours or bodily fluids. These humours were believed to influence a person's physical and mental health, as well as their personality and temperament. The concept of humourism was widely accepted in ancient and medieval medicine and influenced medical practices and beliefs for centuries. Although ideas around exercise, sleep and balance are still important today, luckily draining a person of their bodily fluids to restore balance and promote cheerfulness is no longer considered an appropriate medical practice!

Throughout the journey of seeking to understand autism, some significant mistakes have been made and are still being made. Instead of seeking to understand *why* autistic children use certain behaviours, researchers have stopped at *what*: what are the behaviours, and how shall we change these behaviours? Let me be clear: I am not saying scientific research is bad, but when researching autistic 'ways of being', historically, researchers have taken on the role of judging which human behaviours are deemed appropriate and good and which are deemed inappropriate and bad. But there is another way – autistic researchers and allies are now producing research that recognises and validates autistic traits as valuable and meaningful.

Positive reframing of autistic traits through autistic-led research

'Autism is not behavioural. Atypical behaviour is not autism. It is a consequence of autism. It is surface markers.'[26]

Shannon Des Roches Rosa

Autistic researchers are developing research that reframes autism from a deficit or problem to a divergence or difference. This is an important shift: autistic children should not be considered broken humans. The paperwork that follows autistic children often talk of deficits, delays and disorder; this includes their diagnosis and Education Health Care Plans (plans describing the support disabled children can access in education). The term autism spectrum disorder (ASD) is still used during diagnosis and is even displayed on posters about autistic children. There is much research on how words can impact children's well-being and

26   Rosa, S.D.R. (2019). Autism Is Not 'Behavioral'. [online]
THINKING PERSON'S GUIDE TO AUTISM. Available at: https://
thinkingautismguide.com/2019/05/autism-is-not-behavioral.html
[Accessed 14 Aug. 2023].

sense of self.[27] [28] Instead of developing a strong, positive self-image, autistic children are having their natural development and 'ways of being' described as *disordered*.

Some people are concerned that by portraying autism as a difference or divergence, we may inadvertently downplay the very real challenges that come with being autistic. Conversely, I feel that autistic individuals, as they engage in further research, have the potential to shed light on and destigmatise the complexities of the autistic experience. Whether speaking, pre-speaking or non-speaking, the autistic experience makes it harder to thrive in our society. I am not questioning that. We live in a fast-paced and sensorially busy world, which often has a negative impact on autistic children and adults. It can be disabling. Autistic people are also disabled through current systems and structures that do not prioritise autistic 'ways of being'. In some instances, the autistic person's ability to enjoy a fulfilled life is impacted by internal processes and external factors outside of their own control. But no human should be made to feel like they are broken or that their natural way of developing is flawed, disordered or less than that of other humans.

27   Lodge, J., Harte, D.K. and Tripp, G. (1998). Children's Self-Talk Under Conditions of Mild Anxiety. Journal of Anxiety Disorders, 12(2), pp.153–176. doi:https://doi.org/10.1016/s0887-6185(98)00006-1.

28   Richter, M., Eck, J., Straube, T., Miltner, W.H.R. and Weiss, T. (2010). Do words hurt? Brain activation during the processing of pain-related words. Pain, 148(2), pp.198–205. doi:https://doi.org/10.1016/j.pain.2009.08.009.

The labels we give to children and adults can profoundly impact how others in society view them and how they view and value themselves. Autistic children, no matter their individual divergence, should be afforded the right to be respected and described positively, just as every other child in society has that right.

Deficit-based descriptions of autistic traits can lead others in society to view autistic children less favourably than their peers. Society chooses which humans to invest their time and resources into. It is useful to understand this because, without personal experience of being autistic, the people choosing what to fund may not see autistic requirements as important. It is also likely they will not be impacted by the difficulties autistic families face in trying to adhere to systems and structures that are not built for them.

The following analogy helps to explain how a deficit-based narrative can lead to ableism which impacts people not served by a system. Imagine we live in a world where the majority of children and adults have the ability to fly. Over seven billion people fly around with no need for cars, roads or pavements. Now imagine there are still millions of people who cannot fly, and they *are* in need of cars and roads and pavements, but the powerful players in society will not fund these things as *they* have no need for such things. In this world, school subjects are built around flying, jobs are based on flying, and walkers have to try to fit in as best they can.

The walkers' needs for pavements, roads and cars are

labelled as special needs, and their inability to fly is framed as them having lesser abilities. Powerful players in society, such as governments made up of people who can fly, decide what reasonable adjustments they are willing to make for the walkers. Instead of investing in the structures and systems that the walkers need, money is invested in research and therapies to help these people learn to fly. Try as they might, the children and adults who are walkers simply cannot learn to fly, or if they do, it is incredibly difficult for them, and so they struggle through life as best they can with very few of the necessary resources or adjustments that they need.

From this analogy, we can see how the people in power usually sit within systems that have served them. This is not the case for many families of autistic children. People in power have control over how many resources and how much financial support is afforded to autistic children, their families and their support system. The infrastructure to support autistic children and adults is not just *lacking* in the UK – it is *woefully* lacking and underfunded. A vast amount of money is currently ploughed into autism research, which seeks to 'cure' autism, and into therapies based on changing autistic behaviours to fit an expected pattern. This is instead of money being allocated to help the autistic community thrive, such as developing autistic-friendly schools and targets. Many autistic adults say most current research does not represent their experiences. But there is hope; autistic people are conducting new, progressive research projects. These are focused on explaining how autistic people experience the world and how best to support individual divergence.

Some of the theories that autistic people have developed are:

- The theory of Neurodiversity[29]: This describes cognitive functioning which diverges from the typical or expected functioning. The neurodiversity movement emerged during the 1990s, aiming to increase acceptance and inclusion of all people while embracing neurological differences.

- The Double Empathy Problem[30]: A concept that highlights the bidirectional nature of empathy It addresses the difficulties that arise when autistic and non-autistic individuals try to understand each others' perspectives.

- Monotropism[31]: This refers to a cognitive and attentional style characterised by a strong, singular focus of attention which can lead to complex and detailed learnings.

(These are covered in more detail in *Part Three: Neurosensory Divergence.*)

---

29   Singer, J. (2017). Neurodiversity: the birth of an idea. Lexington, Kentucky: Amazon.

30   Milton, D. (2012). On the ontological status of autism: the 'double empathy problem'. Disability & Society, 27(6), pp.883–887. doi:https://doi.org/10.1080/09687599.2012.710008.

31   Murray, D., Lesser, M. and Lawson, W. (2005). Attention, monotropism and the diagnostic criteria for autism. Autism, 9(2), pp.139–156. doi:https://doi.org/10.1177/1362361305051398.

Building on these theories, this book will explore the new concept of Neurosensory Divergence, which goes beyond behaviours to autistic experiences. Deciphering the internal processes that take place is key to truly understanding autistic traits. I believe sensory divergence (a sensory system that diverges from the expected) is the missing part of the autism story, and it can help us get to those underlying processes.

I have often wondered why the sensory aspects of the autistic profile are still so under-researched, especially when it is one of the most discussed subjects within autistic spaces. One reason could be that people who do not experience sensory divergence simply cannot imagine how important and all-encompassing it is. It is seen as a small part of the autistic profile that may create some challenges. This description downplays one of the most important parts of the human experience: our sensory experiences.

PART TWO:
LIVED EXPERIENCE OF SENSORY DIVERGENCE

In this section, we will explore how experiencing the world through a sensory system that differs from the majority makes life experiences palpably different. Here, the story of sensory divergence is told through a variety of autistic voices, which illuminates how sensory divergence can alter communication and developmental trajectories.

From birth, many autistic children access sensory inputs in ways that are not well understood. In other divergent sensory profiles (such as being deaf or partially deaf), sensory access is understood to stem from neurological or biological divergence. Autistic sensory access is currently framed differently. In autistic children, their divergence is framed as a sensory processing issue they need to overcome through potentially harmful therapy. The description of flawed processing does not align with autistic rich accounts of sensory experiences and many autistic people do not identify with the current framing.

Lived Sensory Experiences

Autistic people are best placed to explain their own autistic experiences. It is important to acknowledge that non-autistic individuals may sometimes struggle to fully empathise with the sensory experiences unique to autism. They may unintentionally minimise the experience of the autistic child. For example, if an autistic child is sensitive to touch and bangs their hand then cries out in pain, people might say, 'That didn't hurt,' or, 'You're okay, that wasn't so bad.' If an autistic child screams because of a bell ringing a person might say, 'There's no need to scream, that wasn't so loud.' These things are often said with well-meaning intentions because the non-autistic person may assume that the autistic child is experiencing the sensory world in the same way as them, but this is not the case for lots of children. Autistic self-reports are full of descriptions identifying the richness and intensity of their autistic sensory experiences.

Rose is an autistic young person who has written a book[32] with her mother, Jodie Smitten, an autistic advocate. Rose discusses her sensory profile, which includes sensations she finds distressing, like 'itchy clothes, such as tights.' She also describes sensory experiences that she enjoys, like "loose-fitting clothing and rollercoasters." When discussing touch, Rose mentions that she finds anyone touching her to be a

---

32   Smitten, R. (2021). The secret life of Rose: inside an autistic head. PP 20-22

peculiar sensation, often prompting her to 'wipe away' the feeling. She does not like hugs or kisses because they don't feel nice to her; she describes them as feeling too tingly. But it is not as simple as thinking that some sensory inputs are bad and others are good. For instance, Rose will give someone a high-five, a type of touch that she is comfortable with. She also explains that loud sounds can make her ears feel like they will explode. Yet she also likes making noise, stating that being loud can be exciting or can help her get her energy out.

Jules is an autistic adult, here she discusses her need for visual stimulation when she was a child:

I never felt like things were colourful enough, bright enough, or vibrant enough in this country. When I visited India, I found I was so stimulated visually because of all the colour, and all of my senses were stimulated, which was so joyful. Creating visual order has always been very pleasurable for me. I like organising things into order. As a child, I was also very artistic.

Jules says that her sensory profile has definitely shaped her adult life, first as a photographer and now as a garden designer.

Leah, an autistic child, explains how her sensory channels of sound and vision seem to work together to help her when playing musical instruments.

Sounds take on colours for me; I always thought it was the same for everyone. I play a few musical instruments, and one day, I said to my teacher, why is the note D purple? He looked so confused and asked what I meant. When I explained that all notes have a different colour, he looked up synaesthesia online, and we read all about it together. It blew my mind that other people cannot see colourful notes!

As these examples show, autistic sensory experiences are varied and complex. Currently, autistic children are often described as being hyper- or hypo-reactive to sensory input. In reality, these experiences can be much more nuanced.

Sensory experiences are not currently considered highly important in the diagnostic criteria. They are described only in terms of a child's behavioural responses to sensory input, with the goal being to reduce sensory divergence. In my opinion, this description only considers the tip of the iceberg. It is based on the observable behaviours and responses which non-autistic people can see. Non-autistic people cannot *see* internal sensory experiences, and this means there can be a lack of understanding and empathy when autistic children struggle with sensory input. The goal of reducing divergence may also be problematic. Although reducing sensory trauma through aids such as noise-cancelling headphones can be helpful, changing autistic sensory profiles may not be either possible or helpful. As both Leah's and Jules's experiences show, divergent sensory experiences can lead to important life skills. It is also important to state that sensory divergence is a spectrum; not everyone will experience the profound sensory experiences discussed above, but even subtle differences in a sensory profile can alter lived experiences.

Recently, an increased understanding that autistic children have sensory divergence *has* fed into some useful supports in schools. These include altering environments to reduce sensory overload, the introduction of sensory rooms, and access to time out of the class to regulate. These supports are commendable and should be considered the gold standard when it comes to sensory supports, but there is so much more to sensory divergence. On an extremely simplistic level, what we access through our senses (input) determines what we learn and, therefore, what we express (output).

Sensory input = sensory output

My interest lies in what autistic children access through their senses, how this information feeds into their neurodiversity, and how it might alter autistic output.

Sensory divergence and communication

When I was teaching, it was obvious that some children in my classroom were experiencing their sensory life differently from their similarly aged peers. Some children would sit quietly exploring how an item looked or felt, and only occasionally, tentatively, would they look up at the children around them who were busily playing together.

Often, these children would have few words and would be flagged as having delayed speech. Although there is consensus that many autistic children face communication challenges, little progress has been made as to why that might be. The words of Donna Williams[33], an autistic author, were a real lightbulb moment for me. In her book, she discusses how she heard words until the age of three. She talks of voices just being a pattern of sound which were like 'a mumbling jumble'.

Donna's descriptions imply that she was accessing words in a strikingly different way than most children access words at the age of three. Although Donna used echolalia (the repetition of sounds or words), she simply wasn't connecting to words conceptually (the words were a pattern of sounds rather than a spoken code with meaning attached); when she repeated words, she was simply repeating a pattern of sounds. One could be forgiven for assuming that Donna was, therefore, not making the cognitive connections needed to understand spoken words. But Donna was building her knowledge in different ways. Although she accessed speech later than her peers, she became an avid reader earlier than many of her peers. She became a writer, artist, singer-

33   Williams, D. (1999). Nobody Nowhere: the remarkable autobiography of an autistic girl. London: Jessica Kingsley.

songwriter, screenwriter, and sculptor. There was just something about Donna's speech access that differed from the majority. Instead of connecting to words, Donna was immersed in the sensory world around her. Many autistic adults recount similar experiences in their childhood, of being disconnected from spoken words and instead attaching meaning to other aspects within their environment.

This idea of sensory access altering a child's learning trajectory is not discussed in relation to autism. As a teacher, I never questioned the steps we took when a child first presented with speech 'delays'. They would be referred for a hearing test, and then, if that came back without pinpointing a hearing issue, they would be referred for a speech and language assessment; if delayed speech sat alongside social differences to the 'expected', the child would be referred for an autism diagnosis. This process was followed on the basis of observable traits but did not investigate why. Questions we could have asked instead were: Why and how is this child accessing speech in a way that diverges from the majority? What communication are they currently using instead? How could we further scaffold the method they *are* using to communicate?

Not accessing speech at an 'expected' age is always framed as bad; children are expected to 'catch up' or risk falling behind. Mainstream schooling systems often struggle to adequately support those who need a different communication method altogether. In the mainstream system, children who cannot access speech or are minimally speaking are often deemed less cognitively able. I have seen this myself. Parents are informed their child is not achieving early learning goals and an assumption is made that the child is struggling academically: but what if they are actually struggling due to sensory divergence with accessing the medium in which those concepts are being taught?

The parents of children who are non- or minimally speaking report that they are often told, by experts and therapists, about all the things their child will *not* achieve. This is coupled with the fact that sensory divergence and delayed access to meaningful communication can result in coping strategies and traits, which are often hard for the speaking and non-sensory divergent community to understand. When a child shows unexpected speech and play traits, assumptions can be made that there is an issue with the parenting. Parents of autistic children are often given conventional advice around speech and play and may even be sent on parenting courses to learn how to play and speak with their child.

Here, Millie (a late diagnosed autistic mother to an autistic child) describes one such scenario:

When my son was three, we were playing at a mud kitchen. I saw another mother and her son playing together. I noticed her son was using lots of rich talk with his mum about what foods they would cook and how yummy they would be. My son was happily opening and closing doors and playing with the kitchen in a minimally verbal way. This was how he always played – he was joyfully parallel playing, paying little attention to me or the other children around him.

My son was first referred for his autism diagnosis a few months later, and I retold this story to the paediatrician observing my son. I explained how my son liked to play, and she replied with the following:

'You really need to try to engage your child by making eye contact and modelling the play. Just use lots of talking about the play.'

Her answer left me feeling inadequate. I knew all of the things she had said – I had modelled language for my son throughout his childhood. He just wasn't interested in playing with his kitchen in that way.

A year or so later, when he began speaking, I listened to his little monologues about his play. I realised that he had always been playing in an exploratory way, discovering in a meaningful way for him. He was looking at the mechanism of the door and seeing what force he needed to use to close and open the door. He was learning and did not need words to learn all the wonderful things he was learning.

(Millie, mother to Luca)

Children with minimal speech often need to use their bodies to communicate their wants and needs; this can include gestures, crying, throwing things and vocalisations. Autistic children often experience sensory overwhelm, and because of the lack of understanding around these experiences, being minimally speaking and unable to explain means that autistic children are extremely vulnerable and may need to use body communication to feel safe. A setting full of noisy, unpredictable children who are all communicating with one another will probably feel very alien, isolating and confusing to a child who is not accessing speech.

Body communication and behaviours that are deemed challenging often elicit the most judgement from others.

When my daughter joined nursery, she would throw things, take toys from other children, pinch other children, and when she was told off, she would bang her head or squeeze herself into a tight space. It was distressing, and I had no idea what to do. The nursery staff tried, but they just found her too challenging and would call me to pick her up. [They] eventually said it was not the correct setting for her, so we ended up with no nursery placement for her.

(Sam, mother to Ollie)

Research suggests a link between reduced access to meaningful communication and certain behaviours deemed challenging. This has always been considered the underlying cause when deaf children display behaviours that challenge. When I read about the history of the deaf community, I became even more convinced that the way autism has traditionally been framed (as a deficit and cognitive disorder) is history repeating itself around a poorly understood neurological and sensory divergence.

Historically, deaf people who could not use spoken language or who accessed delayed spoken language, were deemed cognitively less able. Communication interventions for deaf communities used to focus on developing speech. Those who found speech challenging to access were described as experiencing communication deprivation and were considered lost causes. Without a useful communication tool, many deaf children displayed behaviours such as aggression, emotional distress and avoidance. Alongside this, they also used echolalia and literal thinking and had differences in their executive functioning, understanding of inference, and in their gross and fine motor skills. This list may appear quite familiar, as it encompasses many of the same behaviours typically associated with the autism diagnosis.

Before deaf people devised any official sign languages, many relied on non-speech-based vocalisations such as grunts and gesturing (just as many non- or minimally speaking autistic children do now). In 1817, a deaf man named Laurent Clerc co-founded the first deaf school in America. As his teachings spread, the sign language used in his school combined with other signs from deaf communities to create American Sign Language.

As signing became more prevalent, others in society realised that deaf people were not less cognitively able; in fact, many of them were gifted in specific areas (such as visual memory). Deaf people built community and connection through their signed communication in a way they could not with the non-signing world. Jokes, gossip and inference were all based on deaf knowledge of the world, which is explicitly different from conventional speech-based understanding of the world. Access to useful communication and communities with shared experiences became key to the well-being of deaf children and adults. The deaf community was subsequently viewed as a group of people who could 'create lives based on a different sensory universe than those around them'.[34]

Ido Kedar is an autistic, minimally-speaking author who discusses this subject in his book *Ido in Autismland*.[35] He explains how he was helped to access a useful communication system via a letter board (an alphabet board he could point to), which led to him being able to type. His teacher, Soma Mukhopadhyay, always assumed competence and believed that most students could access meaningful communication with the correct tools. Prior to Ido accessing the letter board and typing, he felt the frustrations of being seen as unaware of the

---

34   Murray, J.J. (2014). History of the deaf. In: Encyclopædia Britannica. [online] Available at: https://www.britannica.com/science/history-of-the-deaf.

35   Ido Kedar (2012). Ido in Autismland: climbing out of Autism's silent prison.

world around him. He sat listening to experts explaining what was wrong with him, while inside, he wanted to tell them they had it all wrong. His therapists stuck to the theories that painted autistic people as having deficits in cognition, and he often felt infantilised. But he was far from childlike. Ido had always been building his own conceptual knowledge of the world, and his mind was rich with insights which were only apparent to others once he had a useful communication tool.

Ido spent a semester at Gallaudet College, a deaf institution of higher education. He reflected on being immersed in a non-speech-based environment:

Associating with deaf people showed me that speech is not a reflection of an intact or intelligent mind but that the human being, if unable to access communication in the conventional verbal pathway, must have another way to express himself.

(Kedar, p18)

Ido's experiences are specific to autistic people who have challenges coordinating their motor skills (often described as verbal apraxia). Ido could hear words and was building his knowledge of the world but could not express this through speech due to his motor constraints. Donna Williams describes a subtly different experience of being autistic, stating she could coordinate her responses to form echolalic scripts. Still, as a young child, she was not assigning meaning to those words. She was instead focused on the sensory inputs around her, which, like Ido's, were at times mesmerising and, at other times, overwhelming. Autistic sensory profiles are complex. In some instances, accessing the world in this way can be both a hindrance and a helpful trait.

This chapter prompts us to ask: Does sensory divergence alter how autistic people acquire language? And if so, how does this impact communication? There have been many opportunities throughout history to reframe autism as a difference that society could accommodate. We are now at a turning point where more and more autistic people are telling their stories. Society can and should be enabling autistic people to 'create lives based on a different sensory universe than that of those around them'.[36]

How sensory aspects of autistic profiles are currently understood

Sensory Integration was first identified as a clinical condition by Anne Ayres in the 1960s (her theory is still used today under the name Sensory Processing Disorder). Ayers was an American occupational therapist and educational psychologist. Her approach is based on the premise that the majority of people are

---

36   Murray, J.J. (2014). History of the deaf. In: Encyclopædia Britannica. [online] Available at: https://www.britannica.com/science/history-of-the-deaf.

born with the ability to manage sensory information, organise it and respond suitably.[37] This is unlike autistic brains, which Ayers said neurologically process sensory stimuli inappropriately, leading to inappropriate behavioural responses. As with other autism theories, it was developed through the deficit-based model and assumes that sensory divergence is a problem that lies within autistic brains. Ayres advocated for sensory integration practices, which (in theory) were supposed to reconfigure autistic neurology to process sensory stimuli in an 'expected' way. Ayres hypothesised that exposing a person to sensory input would help them in a process called sensory gating, where repeated exposure reduces responses.

Imagine if you went to a therapist who said: Because you find it painful when someone sticks a pin in your skin, we are going to slowly introduce sticking pins into your skin to help your brain 'get used to' that experience – not only that, but we will repeat this process weekly until you begin to show signs that you no longer respond to the pain. It may indeed have the desired effect of stopping an external behavioural response, as you will quickly learn that the 'unwanted' behavioural response only leads to more pins being stuck in your hand. Greg Santucci, an occupational therapist who experiences sensory sensitivities, states that therapy should not seek to 'de-sensitize' in this way, as forced or coerced

---

37   Anon, (n.d.). What is Sensory Processing? – Sensory Processing. [online] Available at: https://sensoryprocessinghub. humber.nhs.uk/what-is-sensory-processing/.

sensory exposure can cause trauma.[38]

Sensory integration therapy is controversial because of its similarities to exposure therapy and due to the lack of studies proving its effectiveness. Recent research has indicated that this process does not improve autistic sensory gating.[39] A further study has stated the usefulness of sensory integration therapy may actually lie in increasing autistic children's understanding of their own sensory profiles.[40] For example, a child who builds their knowledge around *their* favoured sensory experiences and triggers could better advocate for their own reasonable adjustments. It has been noted that autistic children often struggle to describe their own sensory divergence[41], possibly because it is rarely discussed except to frame it as problematic.

We must question the rhetoric that autistic sensory experiences are inappropriate. Like any sort of

----

38   Santucci, G. (2022). Facebook. (n.d.). Log into Facebook. [online] Available at: https://www.facebook.com/gregsantucciOT/posts/506604037788846.

39   Davies, P.L. and Gavin, W.J. (2007). Validating the Diagnosis of Sensory Processing Disorders Using EEG Technology. American Journal of Occupational Therapy, 61(2), pp.176–189. doi:https://doi.org/10.5014/ajot.61.2.176.

40   Louise Jane Edgington (2014). The Design and Implementation of a New Cognitive Behavioural Therapy (CBT) Based Intervention for the Management of Sensory Experiences in Adolescents with Autism.

41   Jones, R.S.P., Quigney, C. and Huws, J.C. (2003). First-hand accounts of sensory perceptual experiences in autism: a qualitative analysis. Journal of Intellectual & Developmental Disability, 28(2), pp.112–121. doi:https://doi.org/10.1080/136682503100014705b.

experience, sensory experiences can have both a positive and negative impact on autistic people. For example, taking in lots of detail can be both overwhelming and useful.

When I go into a room, I might hear a clock ticking and children playing outside the room. I might hear the wind whistle through the window, and I would notice the place of every object in the room. If I go into a room for the first time, I might become very quiet because I am taking all that in, but by the third or fourth time, it won't be as intense as I will just be checking everything is still the same as it is in my memory. I do have an amazing memory for the things I have seen!

(Leah, autistic child)

Although there are hard aspects to seeing life in such detail, Leah also explains how her sensory experiences are useful to her. Sensory Integration Theory fails to consider how autistic sensory experiences might be serving autistic people.

It has recently been theorised that autistic children show poor sensory filtering of unnecessary sensory stimuli.[42] This theory states that non-autistic people can relegate some sensory information to the background

---

42   Manning, C., Tibber, M.S., Charman, T., Dakin, S.C. and Pellicano, E. (2015). Enhanced Integration of Motion Information in Children With Autism. Journal of Neuroscience, 35(18), pp.6979–6986. doi:https://doi.org/10.1523/jneurosci.4645-14.2015.

while their senses focus on the most important sensory information. This positions non-autistic sensory experiences as optimal and autistic detailed sensory experiences as problematic.

Many autistic individuals do not describe themselves using the idea that they have a sensory processing disorder or any sort of sensory filtering deficit. Rather, they feel they are accessing *more* sensory input than most people. Therefore, filtering out becomes more challenging. Rachel Wren[43], an autistic consultant, shares her own perspective on current autism theories on social media. Discussing sensory experiences, Wren asserts that she does not have problems filtering; she simply takes in more data through her senses than non-autistic people. She states she does not have slower sensory processing; she just has more sensory data to sort through.

The Sensory Processing Disorder theory alongside research on filtering deficits have added to the narrative that autistic sensory responses are problematic and should be changed. When taking an inside-out approach to autistic sensory experiences, it is quite another story. Instead, it may be the case that autistic children process sensory information in a manner that is useful to them, a manner that society has yet to fully comprehend.

43   TikTok. (n.d.). Auticulate on TikTok. [online] Available at: https://www.tiktok.com/@auticulate/video/7022581512759512325?_r=1&_t=8f1JtlaqyLR [Accessed 21 Aug. 2023].

PART THREE:
NEUROSENSORY DIVERGENCE

The framing of autistic sensory divergence as a flawed processing issue does not seem to explain the rich and tangible sensory experiences that autistic people themselves describe. It does not talk about the way autistic children use sensory information to build knowledge and to demonstrate their inner world. Autistic knowledge is often discounted and overlooked by others because it falls outside of traditional and expected knowledge. In this section, we will explore how autistic children build knowledge, meaning and communication through their own unique sensory profiles.

Neurosensory Divergence: children's experiences

Very early in my teaching career, I had an autistic child in my class called Tommy, who was non-speaking. I had received very little training in supporting autistic children. During my course, we had half a day of instruction on special educational needs[44]*, which I now realise was completely inadequate. When I started teaching Tommy, the school explained that I should assist support staff to ensure Tommy had the resources to access lessons. The Learning Support Assistant (LSA) supporting Tommy had little previous training in supporting non-speaking autistic students. Even the Special Educational Needs Coordinator (SENCO), responsible for overseeing Tommy's access and support, had received minimal training in assisting autistic children.

Here, I would like to state that some of the best, most dedicated and supportive people I have met are Learning Support Assistants (LSAs) and SENCOs. Due to the lack of adequate training, many invest their own time and resources into learning more about the children they are working with. In a bid to support Tommy as best I could, I spent many hours online trying to gain a basic understanding of different types of communication

---

44   * *I dislike the term 'special educational needs' as it assumes that the child needs special treatment when they may actually require a different style teaching. I would much prefer 'learning accessibility adjustments' or learning enrichment.

systems that might work for an autistic child; these included Makaton[45] (a signing language for children) and Picture Exchange Communication[46] (where the child uses pictures to communicate). I created different resources for Tommy so he could access classroom learning.

I noticed very quickly that he was a talented mathematician, and I began to wonder how he had picked up these skills. Was he accessing learning from conversations and teaching, or had he embedded this learning by observing the world around him? I was keen to involve him in lessons by giving him the resources to solve complex maths problems, which he did with very little effort. However, in other lessons, it was hard to know how much of the lesson input he was taking in. It was often assumed that he was not accessing much but that it was nice to include him as much as possible. I have encountered this attitude many times, where a lack of speech has been equated with a lack of ability. However, Tommy's advanced maths skills countered the idea that he was cognitively unable to access learning.

My early interactions with Tommy began to shape my thinking about autism. Tommy appeared to be a happy, bright child who enjoyed being with his peers at

---

45   makaton.org. (n.d.). History - The Makaton Charity. [online] Available at: https://makaton.org/TMC/TMC/The_Makaton_ Charity/A_brief_history_of_Makaton.aspx.

46   Bondy, A. and Frost, L. (2017). Picture Exchange Communica- tion System (PECS)® |. [online] Pyramid Educational Consultants UK. Available at: https://pecs-unitedkingdom.com/pecs/.

times but would also often happily withdraw from other children to investigate textures in the playground. He was overwhelmed by noise at times and yet, at other times, laughed so loudly at his own hidden jokes it would make me jump. This little mathematician in my classroom did not fit any of the stereotyped descriptions of an autistic child. Having the privilege of teaching Tommy made me consider how non- or minimally speaking autistic children may be 'able' in ways that fall outside the expected.

I had many conversations with his parents, who told me that he was very sociable at home with his sister, and they were confused about how rarely he chose to be with his classmates at playtime. I now know that the way an autistic child interacts at home can be hugely different from their presentation at school. For this reason, the insights of parents of autistic children should be valued and believed. Teaching Tommy made me even more interested in how young children learn. While still teaching, I studied the psychology of learning, the particulars of reading acquisition and how babies and children develop language.

Later in my career, I became an early years teacher. My experiences there further reinforced the idea that some children's learning profiles differed significantly from their peers, which seemed to be somehow linked to their sensory profiles. Some children were noticeably struggling in our nursery setting: they cried, held on to their key workers, covered their ears, and spoke very little. I heard these children described as overly attached, clingy, or as school refusers. However, their parents reported that those same children were happy at home in a quiet environment and loved learning and interacting. For other children, the exact opposite was true; at nursery, they seemed quiet and subdued, yet at home (after their day at nursery), they became overwhelmed and frustrated, displaying behaviours that challenged those around them. The link seemed to be that these children were experiencing the sensory world in a way that was not well understood.

The year I started teaching in the Early Years setting, my nephew Jay also started at the same school, in the nursery downstairs from my classroom. It was lovely because I got to see his smiling face every morning. It was also eye-opening because I could see his personality change entirely in the two settings, home and nursery. Jay was engaged with the adults around him at home; he interacted happily and was interested in toys and playing. His home play often centred around programmes he watched, copying phrases from Thomas the Tank Engine as he played with his trains. However, in the nursery, he presented as essentially non-speaking: he watched other children interacting and mostly stayed on the periphery of their interactions. He would play in the playground with a select few other children. Interestingly, the children he really gelled with were also minimally speaking and seemed sensitive to their environment.

Jay was well-liked by his teachers and other children, and he loved being at the nursery, but he could also become distressed at the busy nature of it. His family had already noticed that Jay was sensitive to environments. As a young child, he became distressed when he visited the barber – even the barber holding his hair seemed painful. He also found busy, noisy environments overwhelming and would either shout out, cover his ears or run away. His behaviours may have appeared 'challenging' to outsiders, but these were tangible experiences for Jay and required patience and reassurance. These sensitivities meant he was sometimes anxious as a toddler, startling at unexpected noises such as hand dryers and crying when the sun shone in his eyes.

Jay passed conventional hearing and sight tests. In fact, he was marked out as having exceptional hearing and sight. He seemed to be able to quickly hone in on patterns and items of interest to him. Jay's experiences made me wonder if he could hear more and see more than his peers. However, he also seemed to struggle to hear voices in busy places (like the nursery) where there was a lot of background noise. He would not engage much with formal lessons at nursery and instead was easily distracted by other things that piqued his interest.

Jay's inability to sustain focus in lessons and his lack of interaction and speech at nursery were assumed, by some, to stem from a lack of cognitive ability. However, it was not the case that Jay lacked the ability to learn. Jay had recognised written letters and written words before he could speak fluently; yet he developed speech later than many of his peers and used more echolalia.

Jay has gone on to prove that his cognitive abilities were never impaired, as I will discuss later. However, he has always presented with a spiky learning profile, and this divergence was seen by many as a problem because Jay did not slot easily into the expectations put upon him. Jay seemed to be accessing different learned patterns from his peers. He wasn't picking up on the 'expected' spoken and social patterns and was, therefore, not following the same learning trajectory.

Neurodiversity versus Neurosensory Divergence

I first accessed a useful framework for fully understanding divergent learning trajectories when I studied for my master's degree at Sheffield Hallam University. Their autism course is delivered through autistic tutors and allies (people who respect autistic ways of being). Their teaching was progressive and gave me the tools to begin to understand divergence on a deeper level. The most useful framework to explain this idea of 'different, not less[47]' was *neurodiversity*. A term coined by sociologist Judy Singer, the theory of neurodiversity normalises different ways of thinking and being, positioning brain diversity as a natural occurrence. A person who is neurodivergent has a brain that diverges significantly from the expected or majority,

47   Grandin, T. (2020). Different? Not Less. Future Horizons.

including people who are ADHD, autistic, dyslexic, etc.

This theory was extremely helpful in reframing the autistic experience as divergent from the expected but just as valid. Other theories really stood out in explaining how current perceptions of autistic inner worlds have historically been framed through a non-autistic lens. It was exciting to have access to the latest research by autistic people and their allies, especially as the different theories helped to build a more robust description of autistic profiles.

Three useful theories

Below, I describe three theories which resonated deeply with my understanding of autistic children.

Autistic people have been traditionally described as lacking empathy. Damien Milton's double empathy problem[48] debunks this, suggesting that when people with very different experiences of the world interact with one another, they will struggle to empathise with each other and that this is likely to be exacerbated because of differences in language use and comprehension.

---

48   Milton, D. (2012). On the ontological status of autism: the 'double empathy problem'. Disability & Society, 27(6), pp.883–887. doi:https://doi.org/10.1080/09687599.2012.710008.

Luke Beardon's cross-neurological theory of mind[49] delves into how the majority of people with similar knowledge of the world and similar experiences can mostly infer what that majority is thinking and can, therefore, build lives around that majority's thinking. In the case of autistic children, they fall outside of this and so have less access to systems and supports which serve their requirements.

Finally, monotropism[50], a concept developed by Dinah Murray, Wenn Lawson and Mike Lesser, counters the idea that restricted interests are a negative part of the autistic profile. Instead, this theory states that autistic people tend to have monotropic minds that sustain focus and detailed attention on a small number of interests.

Accessing these theories through my master's helped to explain autistic experiences in a much more comprehensive way, but it still did not feel like the whole story. The focus on neurodivergence was illuminating and intriguing, but it did not explicitly explain sensory experiences. In my experience, sensory experiences are front and centre in most autistic children's everyday lives. For many years, this phenomenon has been left unexplored, even though sensory divergence has

---

49   Beardon, L. (2008). 'Is Autism really a disorder part two – theory of mind? Rethink how we think'. Journal of Inclusive Practice in Further and higher Education, 1: 19 – 21

50   Murray, D., Lesser, M. and Lawson, W. (2005). Attention, monotropism and the diagnostic criteria for autism. Autism, 9(2), pp.139–156. doi:https://doi.org/10.1177/1362361305051398.

run through the narrative surrounding autism since the days of Eugene Bleuler. Traditionally, the sensory aspect in autistic profiles has been discussed only as a small part of autistic 'ways of being'. It has been framed as a divergence that mostly happens in the brain, an inappropriate response to sensory stimuli and something of an add-on to the autism profile. Yet, it is through our senses that we access everything we know. It builds into our conceptual knowledge of the world around us. If autistic children were experiencing sensory input tangibly differently, wouldn't this also impact their learning trajectory?

Some years ago, I was told a story about a six-year-old autistic child who was watching a film with her parents. Halfway through the film, she pointed to a building and said, 'That house is in a strange place, Mummy.' Her parents stared, baffled, as they could not see the house she was pointing to. The girl insisted she could see a house. Her mother checked and was amazed to read that this house had been in the film but had been edited out during postproduction. This little girl had such acute eyesight that she could still see the house that had been edited out! The same year, I was travelling in the car with my nephew Jay, and two of his friends. As we drove along, Jay (who was by that time identified as autistic) shouted, 'Let it go, let it go!' The other children in the car and I were slightly perplexed by Jay suddenly bursting into song. Then he said, 'I love this song.' I replied, 'The radio isn't on,' but he insisted, 'Yes, it is – turn it up!' Sure enough, when I turned it up, *Let It Go* sang out from the radio! I told Jay he had amazing ears.

These stories do not make sense if we think of autistic auditory or visual sensory experiences as a processing difference or as a case of filtering information in and out. These children seemed to see and hear *more*.

Jay's acute hearing had been with him since he was born. He didn't sleep through the night as he was woken by cars, planes and noises in the street. He cried at the hairdryer and the vacuum cleaner and was easily startled by loud noises. He was a happy, giggly baby, but his mother was told there were issues with his development: his speech was delayed, which indicated he might be autistic. He was indeed identified as autistic.

Over time, his sensory sensitivity has changed and settled. But his acute hearing means he can now play the piano by ear. This is even more interesting when you consider that no one in his house is musical and he had not been around anyone musical. Jay also developed other skills that seemed to materialise innately, without too much teaching input. It appeared that when Jay had access to meaningful resources, he was a little sponge learning patterns of numbers, letters and musical notes. Yet he was judged as being 'behind' his peers in many conventional skills such as self-feeding, dressing, speaking and listening. You may wonder why a child with such acute hearing had delayed speech – I will come on to that later.

Jay's developmental journey got me thinking. I had always subscribed to sociology's teachings around nurture, where emphasis is placed on the role of the parents, teachers and peers in moulding children's abilities and talents. However, it appeared that Jay's natural ability to play music and tune into patterns of learning, which sat outside the 'expected', was somehow linked to his sensory divergence. Instead of accepting the current narrative, I thought about why sensory divergence occurs and how it might appear in autistic developmental profiles.

Neurosensory Divergence: an inside-out explanation

To explain divergent developmental profiles, looking at both neurological and physical internal processes is useful. We start life with a brain that is a sort of unique blueprint of neural pathways created through our parents' and ancestors' learnings and experiences. This does not mean we are born with their abilities and knowledge, but that we may have inherited some of their hardware (brain structures), and this can impact what we learn and how we learn from our environment. Not only can we add to these neural connections, we can also forge novel connectivity through neuroplasticity. This means that we do not all learn and process information in the same way as one another; this is called neurodiversity. This phenomenon has been used to explain the neurological underpinnings of autistic brains. However, neurodiversity does not extend to the analysis of how the brain and sensory system interact.

We learn about the world by observing patterns around us, translating these through the senses and neurologically generating behavioural responses. This happens when sensory stimuli in the environment activate sensory receptors (on or in our bodies). These receptors convert sensory signals into electrical or chemical signals (sensations). These sensations then travel via nerve fibre to the relevant sensory area of the brain. Neurons then transmit information between brain cells.

Brain connectivity in sensory areas is organised broadly based on function. There is the auditory cortex, which deals with sounds. The visual cortex deals with sight, the gustatory cortex with taste, the sensory cortex with touch, and the olfactory bulbs with smell. Sensory inputs usually travel through the nervous system to specific brain areas. This, in turn, leads the brain to be in a state of 'action potential', where the brain groups the sensory information in the context of pre-existing information and predicts the next course of action. Connections across the brain are then used to make sense of the information. This process of gathering information from the senses can reinforce a person's current concepts or create new conceptual learning. This will be represented in the brain's neural connectivity (the connections in and between brain regions). Autistic brains have been shown to have hyperconnectivity in some areas of the brain and less connectivity in other areas.[51] For example, the hippocampus, which is thought to be involved in language processing and memory, presents with divergent connectivity in some autistic children[52].

So much of learning is a sensory business. The more we access and learn, the more neural connections we make. And if we access different sensory inputs from one another, it stands to reason that we will learn different things from one another and create divergent neural connections from the expected. The brain is interconnected, influenced and altered by other systems in the body. In fact, to think of the brain as a separate entity within the body is problematic; the brain is very much part of the body's ecosystem. This brain-body connection is very apparent when relating this to the body's sensory system. When a specific sense struggles to access some or all sensory information from the environment, this can trigger a sequence of events within the brain that allows other senses to take over.

This rerouting of signals has been noted in deaf people, where auditory deprivation causes the brain to reorganise and increase activity in other senses. This phenomenon has also been observed in partially sighted

51   Kana, R.K., Uddin, L.Q., Kenet, T., Chugani, D. and Müller, R.-A. (2014). Brain connectivity in autism. Frontiers in Human Neuroscience, 8. doi:https://doi.org/10.3389/fnhum.2014.00349.

52   Banker, S.M., Gu, X., Schiller, D. and Foss-Feig, J.H. (2021). Hippocampal contributions to social and cognitive deficits in autism spectrum disorder. Trends in Neurosciences, [online] 44(10), pp.793–807. doi:https://doi.org/10.1016/j.tins.2021.08.005.

and blind individuals, where they are able to isolate sounds with greater acuity. Some blind and deaf people have also been shown to have 'super senses' within their sensory profile, which are senses that effectively do double the work to make up for the less useful sensory areas (throughout this book, I refer to these super senses as *sensory abundance*). Similarly, many autistic people report that they have specific senses (or elements within their senses) that present as super senses, where they appear to be taking in more sensory stimuli.

Vitally, it has now been posited that autistic sensory divergence *can* be a physical experience in some autistic people rather than only being present in the brain. Recent studies have shown that some autistic people hear more[53] [54], as opposed to being unable to filter out noise. Similarly, this phenomenon has been

---

53   Kuiper, M.W.M., Verhoeven, E.W.M. and Geurts, H.M. (2019). Stop Making Noise! Auditory Sensitivity in Adults with an Autism Spectrum Disorder Diagnosis: Physiological Habituation and Subjective Detection Thresholds. Journal of Autism and Developmental Disorders, [online] 49(5), pp.2116–2128. doi:https://doi.org/10.1007/s10803-019-03890-9.

54   Remington, A. and Fairnie, J. (2017). A sound advantage: Increased auditory capacity in autism. Cognition, 166, pp.459–465. doi:https://doi.org/10.1016/j.cognition.2017.04.002.

noted in the visual senses of some autistic people[55] [56] [57], where enhanced perceptual abilities have been recorded.[58] Furthermore, a study focusing on sensitivity to touch found that tactile sensitivities can be present in autistic individuals[59], with another finding that this phenomenon might affect nerves in the skin rather than being down to neurological processing.[60] These studies indicate that sensory divergence (in some autistic people) could be a tangible divergence that is found not only in the brain but also in the sensory organs (ears, eyes, skin, nose and mouth).

55   Brinkert, J. and Remington, A. (2020). Making sense of the perceptual capacities in autistic and non-autistic adults. Autism, 24(7), p.136236132092264. doi:https://doi.org/10.1177/1362361320922640.

56   Grandgeorge M, Masataka N. Atypical Color Preference in Children with Autism Spectrum Disorder. Front Psychol. 2016 Dec 23;7:1976. doi: 10.3389/fpsyg.2016.01976. PMID: 28066297; PMCID: PMC5179595.

57   Samson, F., Mottron, L., Soulières, I. and Zeffiro, T.A. (2011). Enhanced visual functioning in autism: An ALE meta-analysis. Human Brain Mapping, 33(7), pp.1553–1581. doi:https://doi.org/10.1002/hbm.21307.

58   EurekAlert! (n.d.). New research explains autistic's exceptional visual abilities. [online] Available at: https://www.eurekalert.org/news-releases/772309 [Accessed 14 Aug. 2023].

59   Failla, M.D., Gerdes, M.B., Williams, Z.J., Moore, D.J. and Cascio, C.J. (2020). Increased pain sensitivity and pain-related anxiety in individuals with autism. Pain Reports, [online] 5(6). doi:https://doi.org/10.1097/PR9.0000000000000861.

60   Ehrhart, F., Sangani, N.B. and Curfs, L.M.G. (2018). Current developments in the genetics of Rett and Rett-like syndrome. Current Opinion in Psychiatry, 31(2), pp.103–108. doi:https://doi.org/10.1097/yco.0000000000000389.

This muddies the water somewhat when it comes to sensory processing because it moves away from the simplistic view of a neurological sensory processing disorder as the defining reason for autistic sensory traits. Viewing autism as a neurological and sensory divergence gives a much clearer picture of internal processes that can underlie autistic traits. This perspective suggests that the reorganisation of the brain may occur because the sensory system is actively seeking the most relevant sensory information, a process that can vary among autistic individuals. Senses that *can* access a wider range of sensory data may be playing an enhanced role within the sensory systems of autistic individuals. Often, researchers are baffled as to why autistic children, who fall under a single diagnostic label, present with such different neurological and behavioural profiles. Neurosensory Divergence could potentially provide the key to unravelling this mystery.

The concept of tangible sensory experiences marries with the descriptions of so many autistic people I have spoken to, like Jay's explanation of it feeling like needles in his scalp when the hairdresser holds his hair or the student who told me that wires and lights often buzz so loudly she cannot focus in the classroom. It also explains why an autistic child might hear a song when the radio is turned down extremely low or see a building edited out of a film – those children could hear and see more than most people. Temple Grandin, the autistic scientist, echoes this experience, describing her heightened visual acuity and the resulting hyperconnectivity in her visual cortex (further discussed in Part Seven). This phenomenon of autistic sensory abundance is an important area for future research.

It is also important to dispel the idea that exposure therapy is helpful for sensory abundance. Even when sensory divergence is underpinned by neuroplasticity as opposed to biological differences, autistic people cannot just change what they see, hear, feel, taste or touch (as is the aim of sensory integration therapy). Although this type of therapy *could* dampen responses, the risk of traumatising an autistic child seems too great to justify its use. Attempting to undo sensory divergence is probably not optimal for the autistic child, whose profile has grown around that sensory divergence.

Take the cases of Pauline Bleuler, Donna Williams and Anand Prahlad[61], who all experienced different types of synaesthesia, where two or more senses work together to decipher sensory information. All of these people had skills that had probably grown because of their neurosensory divergent profiles. It is probable that their brains and senses reorganised to work in the most efficient manner for their profile. If these people had been treated with acceptance throughout their lives and their sensory divergence believed, supported and validated, it is very probable they would have experienced less trauma. Just as we no longer expect left-handed individuals to become right-handed, the

61   Anand Prahlad (2017). The secret life of a Black Aspie : a memoir. Fairbanks, Ak: University Of Alaska Press.

goal should never be to change an autistic child into a non-autistic child. Instead, I firmly believe that our focus should be on gaining a deeper understanding of sensory profiles to develop and implement valuable and effective support systems.

So why is research into sensory experiences not growing? The issue may be that to test autistic senses, researchers must rely on autistic self-reports of sensory experiences. Historically, researchers have framed autistic children as unreliable reporters of their own experiences, meaning researchers have relied instead on phenomena that can be observed. However, a gap exists between observational behavioural studies, which frequently attribute sensory divergence to flawed neurological processes and autistic self-reports, which vividly depict sensory experiences as tangible events.

Many autistic children find it hard to explain exactly what they experience. This could be because of a lack of useful representations of autistic sensory experiences around them in either the media or books. It could also be down to communication barriers. Although communication can present challenges, researching autistic children's sensory experiences *is* possible. A recent study found innovative ways (such as using video clips and storytelling) to help children describe their sensory experiences.[62]

---

62   Kirby, A.V., Dickie, V.A. and Baranek, G.T. (2014). Sensory experiences of children with autism spectrum disorder: In their own words. Autism, 19(3), pp.316–326. doi:https://doi. org/10.1177/1362361314520756.

Often, the children who present with the most pronounced sensory divergence are non-speaking or pre-speaking children, possibly because their neurological, motor and/or sensory profile diverges significantly from the expected, making access to speech more challenging. The inability to see inside their world through spoken conversations creates a barrier to understanding their internal processes. By fostering curiosity about their sensory profiles and embracing their autistic communication cues, along with drawing from accounts of non-speaking or pre-speaking autistic individuals, we can attempt to decipher every autistic child's sensory profile.

Sensory divergence could also be picked up through diagnostic testing. Although sensory deprivation may be picked up through sight and hearing tests, sensory abundance is rarely flagged or supported. It may seem strange to consider sensory abundance a problem, but for many autistic children, sensory abundance can create huge access issues (as we will explore later).

Another issue with researching this phenomenon is that sensory profiles can change over time. This could be partly down to damage to the receptors, as is the case with tinnitus, which many autistic people experience. It could also be due to changes in sensory profiles. For example, sensory abundance might be dampened as children mature.

Why does Neurosensory Divergence exist?

It is important to note that sensory divergence and the resulting traits can present for many different underlying reasons. Some people believe that autism is always hereditary, passed down from parents. This belief has arisen due to the frequent occurrence of parents identifying as autistic once their child is diagnosed as autistic. There is currently a discussion in the autism community about whether *all* autistic children's parents should be assessed for autism. It is essential to recognise that although this may be true for many families, it is not *always* true. Autism may be better understood as an umbrella term encompassing various underlying factors that can create autistic traits.

Autistic traits are the resulting behavioural strategies that autistic people employ as necessary when underlying neurological, sensory or motor divergence is present. Neurosensory Divergence can occur when there is any underlying reorganisation from the expected. In cases of apraxia, where motor divergence makes it challenging to form words, the brain may undergo reorganisation to access alternative communication systems, such as visual or tactile methods. This adaptation could potentially trigger further sensory divergence as the brain compensates for the communication challenges, leading to sensory abundance in the senses that are doing double the work. Sensory deprivation (such as sight or hearing loss) can also trigger neurological reorganisation, resulting in sensory abundance. It is also possible that having a parent or ancestor with hearing or sight loss could predispose children to sensory divergence, such as synaesthesia and sensory abundance, through inherited neurological structures. Additionally, the brain generates new neural activity when a person focuses intensely on a particular interest or when mastering a new skill, and this, too, can manifest as neurological reorganisation and sensory abundance. This process underscores the remarkable adaptability of both the brain and the body to adapt and find alternative ways to access sensory information.

Tom Chi's TED Talk[63] illustrates how sensory focus can alter neurological connections in the brain while simultaneously altering the balance within the body. He explains that if you were to look into the mind of a concert pianist, you would see how much of their brain is dedicated to this instrument. The way the person uses the foot pedal coordinates their fingers on the piano, and their knowledge of music theory would all be retained. This involves not only memory but also muscle memory. It is akin to learning another language, where the person's focus and knowledge of the piano will be represented as different patterns and structures within the brain.

Chi explains that this pattern in the brain was not

63   Everything is Connected -- Here's How: | Tom Chi | TEDxTaipei. (2016). YouTube. Available at: https://www.youtube.com/watch?v=rPh3c8Sa37M.

possible just a few hundred years ago before the piano was invented in the 1700s. It is in this way that neurological hardware passed on can alter neurosensory profiles. His explanation gives a glimpse into how Neurosensory Divergence can be passed from generation to generation simply by being an expert in a field. Neurological structures may well predispose future generations toward picking up certain environmental patterns of learning. This understanding shifts the way we currently think of children's learning; if some children are predisposed to pick up divergent patterns in their environment, then expecting them to fit into expected and conventional patterns of learning is unfair and puts them at a disadvantage.

Both biological and neurological processes are likely involved in the presentation of Neurosensory Divergence. Whether the underlying reason for Neurosensory Divergence is primarily neurological or biological, the result is that many autistic people access sensory inputs divergently because they are seeking out the most useful information for their own neurosensory profile. Autistic children must find their way through life with brains and bodies that do not fit expectations. Existing in a predominantly non-autistic world creates a disconnect between the systems, structures and supports that autistic people need versus the systems, structures and supports that are currently in place to meet non-autistic needs. Reframing some autistic people's experiences through a Neurosensory Divergence lens could prove very useful in rethinking how we support autistic children.

Autistic Neurosensory Divergence (NSD) Definition

Neurosensory Divergence is a biological, physiological, and/or neurological divergence that alters the sensory information that a person can access, assimilate and express. By default, autistic people focus on the most useful sensory inputs based on their own individual neurosensory profile. This can lead to the formation of communication styles, traits and learning profiles that fall outside of expected trajectories.

Co-occurring conditions

There is a chicken-and-egg situation to unpick regarding whether Neurosensory Divergence creates co-occurring conditions or vice versa. These are currently seen as a coincidental element within autistic profiles. However, as I explain below, many co-occurring conditions (or divergences) may be interlinked as part of the underlying reason for autistic traits.

Hypermobility, Ehlers-Danlos syndromes and dyspraxia

Many autistic children are diagnosed with motor conditions (where motor skills diverge from the expected). These include hypermobility, Ehlers-Danlos syndromes (EDS) and dyspraxia. Diagnosed children may develop their motor skills (such as handwriting, potty training and self-dressing) along a different timeline than expected. Autistic children are often pushed to overcome these challenges and 'catch up' with other children their age.

Hypermobility is also linked to multiple sensory differences. For example, hypermobility can alter the maturation process of the middle ear, meaning it can take longer to mature. Hypermobility of the joints can also alter the way sound is conducted. EDS has been shown to trigger progressive and intermittent hearing loss. Hypermobility and EDS have also been linked to sight issues, such as sensitivity to light, convergence (where the eyes are less synchronised) and other ocular differences.

Prevalence of hearing and vision differences

Researchers have found a prevalence of hearing and vision differences in autistic children, including hyperopia (farsightedness), astigmatism (distorted vision), myopia (nearsightedness) and strabismus (a condition where the eyes point in different directions). Additionally, hearing loss is thought to be at least three times as common in autistic children as in the general population.[64] Autistic children may have hearing loss

---

64   Confusion at the crossroads of autism and hearing loss. (2020). Spectrum. [online] 14 Aug. Available at: https://www. spectrumnews.org/features/deep-dive/confusion-at-the-cross roads-of-autism-and-hearing-loss/.

in specific ranges. For example, high-pitched sounds might be very loud, or a child may not hear mid or low-pitched sounds clearly. Such differences cause access barriers to sensory inputs and may be part of some autistic children's NSD profiles.

Attention-Deficit/Hyperactivity Disorder (ADHD)

Many children are diagnosed with both ADHD and Autism. Although ADHD children may display similar traits to autistic children, the underlying neurology and sensory experiences of ADHD children and autistic children might differ considerably. Both ADHD and autistic children may experience sensory access issues, communication divergence, and focus challenges, but these challenges will present in different ways. Autistic children who are diagnosed autistic/ADHD usually present with hyperactivity or challenges focusing alongside autistic traits. ADHD children are more likely to be hyper-polytropic (processing many sensory channels at once), whereas autistic children are likely to be predominantly monotropic (processing singular channels). Although there is overlap, as both ADHD and autistic children can share both monotropic and hyper-polytropic tendencies, the distinction between the two diagnoses could be useful in offering tailored supports.

Trauma

Autistic children can experience ongoing sensory trauma and emotional trauma. Sensory trauma may occur due to overloading and sensorily stimulating environments; emotional trauma may occur due to identity rejection and a lack of societal understanding and support of autistic 'ways of being'. Trauma can also result from a lack of autonomy over autistic unmet needs. Conventional cognitive therapy is often unhelpful as many of the traumas autistic children experience come from external sources and are sustained and ongoing. These experiences can result in anxiety and depression, which can physically impact the body.

Autoimmune and chronic conditions

Autoimmune conditions and allergies are often present in autistic populations. Researchers have found that autoimmune conditions, motor conditions, food allergies, long-term chronic pain conditions, inflammation, gastro conditions and hormonal imbalances often co-occur in individuals who have experienced trauma. This is thought to be because trauma affects the hypothalamic-pituitary-adrenal (HPA) axis, which is thought of as the neuroendocrine link between stress and the body's physiological reaction to stress.

Gut microbiomes have also been shown to become unbalanced when the body is under stress. This means that when a hard-to-process food like gluten or dairy enters the body, this further upsets the gut microbiome. The brain and body have a finite number of resources to allocate to fighting such imbalances. In some people, the body actively rejects some foods and toxins in the form of allergies and auto-immune responses.

All of the above conditions increase the load on autistic brains and bodies, creating a cycle of trauma, brain fog, inflammation and chronic illness in some individuals.

Regressive autism

Where autism presents after specific skills have been acquired and then lost (such as speech and self-care), this indicates further divergence has developed. Physical, neurological, genetic or stress factors can be the cause. In all cases of regressive autism, where the child loses skills, the underlying cause should be investigated. Ongoing regression should not be confused with temporary regression, where the child loses some skills for a period but quickly regains them. This can happen in all children when, for example, they are under extra stress, such as being unwell or tired.

Verbal apraxia

Verbal apraxia (also known as verbal dyspraxia and apraxia of speech) leads to many of the traits seen in NSD autistic children; however, verbal apraxia alters how children use their motor skills to make sounds. With apraxia, not all behaviours should be considered communication, as some verbal sounds and movements may be unintentional. Apraxia and autism can co-occur, but the apraxia element would require different types of supports from neurosensory divergence.

PART FOUR:
SENSORY ACCESS

Sensory access is not often considered with regard to autistic children, but it can change how they learn and interact with their surroundings. Autistic children can experience sensory abundance *and* deprivation within their sensory profiles.

Sensory abundance and the conference effect

Sensory abundance can cause access issues, because taking in more sensory input can make it much harder to access 'expected' sensory inputs. Imagine being in a conference where everyone is talking at once. It makes it much harder to hear the person sitting next to you. You might have to lean in to hear them clearly. This is not a sudden inability to filter out noise. It is lots of noise all happening at once.

Now imagine yourself in a classroom, and all the sounds, sights or smells and so on are 'turned up', so now you can hear the birds singing, the cars outside, the aeroplane overhead, children in the classroom next door, and the wires buzzing; you can see children moving around you and the lights flickering; you can smell the dinner hall smells from downstairs. All these inputs create a conference effect, making it very hard to tune into something like a teacher's voice at the front of the classroom. This is not a problem with filtering but rather an abundance of sensory input. The conference effect should always be considered when autistic children struggle with focus.

Conventional knowledge states that autistic children should not use aids because they need to get used to sounds in order to process those sounds correctly. Although there may be an element of this 'getting used to', which is important, this thinking also leaves some autistic children vulnerable to ongoing sensory trauma instead of investigating whether aids could be helpful for some autistic children.

We trialled a hearing device with my Nephew Jay whereby he wore headphones, and his teacher wore a microphone to amplify her voice. We kept the volume low so as not to distress Jay. The teacher reported that Jay's eyes lit up when he heard her voice, which greatly helped with focus. Our lived experience tells me that there is so much more we can do to support autistic sensory abundance.

Sensory deprivation

Autistic profiles may often include sensory deprivation, where the child struggles to access some sensory information. I recently chatted with a speech and language therapist who said many children with communication and social differences experienced early childhood recurrent ear infections or glue ear infections. A friend of mine, who is autistic, experiences cookie bite hearing, where she experiences mid-range frequency hearing loss. This means she has to focus much more intensely on visual cues. Sensory deprivation should always be investigated alongside sensory abundance when mapping any child's sensory profile.

PART FIVE:

LEARNING PROFILES

Children are always learning, and autistic children are no exception. Due to their Neurosensory Divergence, they may well be less focused on the expected. This means they may be learning things which are entirely unexpected. Considering how autistic children access, assimilate and express sensory information is the key to really understanding autistic children's profiles.

Pattern Recognition as part of learning profiles

Divergent neurosensory profiles are most likely present from birth in many autistic children. That means that long before they are officially identified as autistic, these children often experience the sensory world differently from the majority. Autistic babies use the same process of investigation as the majority. Babies and toddlers constantly observe, copy, categorise and test in order to learn. Only as these babies develop their own traits will differences in how and what they are learning become more noticeable. Autistic babies may be more interested and engaged with objects and exploration as they may not be accessing voices; voices could blend into the cacophony of sensory input around them.

Because of the busy sensory landscape, autistic children will focus on the most useful sensory information for their unique sensory profile. This leads to autistic children having unexpected pattern spotting. Simon Baron-Cohen writes about this phenomenon in his book *The Pattern Seekers*.[65] In this book, he discusses pattern spotting in relation to autistic savants (someone with an extraordinary area of knowledge or ability) and those who accelerated the advancement of human civilisation through their pattern-spotting abilities. Many autistic children can indeed present with sensory abundance, and so may have superior pattern-spotting abilities. But it is also true that *all* babies and children access and copy patterns to learn; it is just that autistic children are privy to patterns that diverge from the expected. An autistic child whose neurology and sensory system is organised to take in information primarily through their sense of touch will experience the world very differently from a child who is learning primarily through their sense of sight.

Let's consider a child who primarily uses their visual

---

65   Baron-Cohen, S. (2020). The Pattern Seekers. Penguin UK.

sense to learn about the world around them. Look around you now. How many visual patterns can you spot in your current environment? As I sit here in my office, I can see a set of drawers that are built in an aesthetically pleasing pattern, bricks in houses that are laid in a pattern to ensure a sturdy structure, lampposts that are spaced equally, and cars parked lined up on a road. Children who cannot use their auditory sense to access the spoken code of speech (which incidentally is also a pattern) might instead be immersed in a world of visual patterns, tactile patterns, or even taste patterns. Depending on which senses are being used, an autistic pre-speaking, minimally speaking, or non-speaking child might be learning a great deal from the patterns around them. The most efficient way they have of communicating that learning is through recreating those visual patterns in their play.

Early exploratory play is often about children observing and recreating the experiences around them. Children who are learning to communicate through speech often recreate what they see and what they hear by acting out scenarios they have experienced. For example, a child might play with a toy vacuum and say the word 'vacuum'. The child is recreating a pattern of behaviour and a code they have noticed. Children who are learning to communicate through their most useful current sense (perhaps their sense of sight or touch) may be noticing different patterns from their peers. They may see patterns and colours more vividly and notice intricate tactile patterns around them. Colour coding toys, lining up items and creating patterns are all forms of exploratory play and communication; feeling textures around the playground or sniffing objects is all exploratory play.

Some people think alternative styles of exploration and play are less useful than expected learning and play. But really, does play ever have to be useful or understood by others? If the child takes joy in what they are exploring, the only viable course of action is undoubtedly to revel in that joy and commend them on the outcome of their exploration. Joining with them in these moments will offer them feedback that what they are doing is important and valid. Alongside this, we have no idea what autistic children are learning when they have minimal ways of communicating it.

Temple Grandin, an autistic scientist, remembers being extremely withdrawn and sensitive to touch and sound as a child. She did not start talking until she was three and a half. Instead, she focused on storing the visual patterns around her as concepts that she pieced together to make meaning. She puts this down to her extraordinary vision, saying she can still spend hours studying tiny pattern variations in a carpet. By the time Temple was seven, her exploratory play looked more like scientific experimentation. She spent hours making parachutes and experimenting with throwing them up in the air; this required careful observation to make slight design changes to make her parachutes work better. She says she was single-minded and focused on the visual information she accessed, and explains that she has always thought in pictures and that words are a second language to her, stating that when someone speaks to her, she translates that speech into pictures. Grandin states that non-autistic people struggle to imagine and understand her internal processes.[66] [67] [68]

People who experience sensory divergence can come up against a society that does not fully understand or believe their experiences. This was the case for a lady called Joy Milne, from Scotland, who experienced a heightened sense of smell. There is nothing to indicate that Joy is autistic (when sensory divergence does not impact communication autism is not usually diagnosed), but like Temple Grandin, she does experience sensory divergence. Twelve years before Joy's husband was diagnosed with Parkinson's disease, Joy noticed a musky smell coming from him. After he was diagnosed, Joy went with him to places where there were other people with Parkinson's and discovered that she smelled that same musky smell on them. She discussed this phenomenon with a scientist who was sceptical,

66   Grandin, T. (2006). THINKING IN PICTURES: Autism and Visual Thought. [online] www.grandin.com. Available at: https://www.grandin.com/inc/visual.thinking.html.

67   Hughes, V. (2009). Autism often accompanied by 'super vision', studies find | Spectrum | Autism Research News. [online] Spectrum | Autism Research News. Available at: https://www.spectrumnews.org/news/autism-often-accompanied-by-super-vision-studies-find/.

68   Grandin, T. (2023). Opinion | Temple Grandin: Society Is Failing Visual Thinkers, and That Hurts Us All. The New York Times. [online] 9 Jan. Available at: https://www.nytimes.com/2023/01/09/opinion/temple-grandin-visual-thinking-autism.html.

assuming such a skill was impossible; they tested Joy to see if she could identify people who were diagnosed with Parkinson's just by smelling their clothes. She could! Joy experiences hereditary hyperosmia (super smell), and her insights have proved invaluable.[69]

Just like Temple and Joy, many autistic children's sensory divergence leads to divergent pattern spotting. There is a lack of understanding around autistic play and pattern recognition, which risks these children's experiences and talents being disregarded or invalidated. Unique and unexpected pattern spotting means that some autistic children will access patterns of learning that the majority simply cannot access. These include things like having perfect pitch, advanced mathematical abilities and the ability to reproduce songs or draw with precision. Autistic pattern spotting may also include the ability to taste, smell or feel things with greater acuity. Autistic play and learning, just like expected play and learning, can lead autistic children to all sorts of interesting discoveries. For example, a child who is invested in exploring the grain in a wooden item or a child who listens to the same sound on repeat is probably learning and embedding in a very meaningful way.

By viewing autism through a developmental lens, we

69   Improving Parkinson's Disease diagnosis. (n.d.). Improving Parkinson's Disease diagnosis. [online] Available at: https://www. manchester.ac.uk/discover/news/a-nose-to-diagnose-improv ing-parkinsons-diagnosis/#:~:text=Joy%20Milne%20is%20a%20 [Accessed 14 Aug. 2023].

can understand that autistic children are learning and growing along their own developmental pathways. Rather than seeing autistic traits as different, it is useful to understand that learning from and recreating patterns is a natural human trait. These traits may appear magnified in autistic children, but they are still very much human. For example, the behaviour of organising the observable into neat categories is a human behaviour that autistic children display when they line up and colour code their toys. This is the same method a scientist might use to categorise different species and chemical elements. It is simply the framing of such traits that creates the concept that in an autistic child, this behaviour is 'abnormal'. Expecting autistic children to move away from their natural self-directed learning takes away their autonomy and their intrinsic drive to learn. Autistic children may not follow an expected learning trajectory. Divergent pattern spotting due to Neurosensory Divergence is a huge part of how autistic profiles develop. The issue here does not lie within the autistic child's development but in the fact that comparing an autistic profile to an 'expected' profile is a flawed method of monitoring autistic children.

Autistic pattern recognition and spiky learning profiles

This concept of Neurosensory Divergence places access to sensory inputs as the most important factor within autistic profiles. Each autistic person can have a different balance of sensory access to another person and, therefore, any combination of pattern recognition. Although there may be groups of autistic traits, the current descriptions of behaviours assumed to sit across *all* autistic people are far too simplistic to capture the complex nature of autism.

The idea of not viewing autistic people as a homogeneous group has recently been presented by a group of developmental cognitive neuroscientists. The team within CALM[70] (The Centre for Attention, Learning and Memory) at Cambridge University used a transdiagnostic research model to study learning profiles. This model acknowledges that the labels used to describe Special Educational Needs, such as autistic or ADHD, are often arbitrarily assigned based on outward behaviours and that, in fact, two children with the same label may have completely different learning profiles. Therefore, the research was not conducted with a cohort of children with one diagnosis (such as autism) but with children who displayed similar traits. The team mapped the learning profiles and brain mechanisms

---

70   Astle, D. E., Bathelt, J., CALM team, & Holmes, J. (2019). Remapping the cognitive and neural profiles of children who struggle at school. Developmental Science, 22(1), e12747.

of 550 children aged five to eighteen who had been referred by health and educational professionals for having traits often associated with learning divergence, such as attention differences, memory challenges, language differences, or poor school progress.

The data the team gathered about the children included assessments of cognitive abilities and MRI scans of the brain. Importantly, this sat alongside questionnaires filled out by the family and child about the child's traits, well-being, family history and communication. This type of multifaceted study is a valuable tool for including lived experience. A useful future approach could be to include studied groups as co-developers in both the design and delivery of the research.

With the information gathered, the team could map each child's abilities and challenges and compare this with their MRI scans. The team had predicted that children with ADHD would present with similar learning profiles and that autistic children would have similar learning profiles. However, this was not the case. The team found that learning profiles did not correlate with the children's diagnoses. For example, one child diagnosed as autistic might have a poor working memory but show abilities in other areas, and another child diagnosed as autistic may have a good working memory but struggle in other areas. The team also found that children with the same diagnoses did not necessarily have the same underlying reason for the divergence seen in their learning profiles. These significant findings indicate that a diagnosis does not tell us very much about each child's unique profile.

Human development is messy, dynamic and constantly evolving. Even divergent traits (including learning profiles) are impacted by internal and external factors, adding to the complexity of divergence itself. Researchers often attempt to reduce the classification of ways of being into a box-ticking exercise where observable traits are grouped together under a diagnosis. Systems and structures built around expected ways of learning discount divergent learning styles, regarding them as problematic, when in reality the systems and structures do not offer true equity within education. Being neurosensory divergent, with sensory abundance, may lead to divergent pattern spotting and spiky learning profiles. But if autistic children are not a homogeneous group, why are there some traits which *are* present in the majority of autistic children? These include meltdowns, shutdowns, stimming and monotropism. The CALM team's neurological mapping and machine learning may hold the key to this question.

Through their research, the team found that, in the cohort of children they were working with, the children's brains were organised in networks connected by hubs. They explained that some presented with large hubs like the big stations in an underground rail map, such as King's Cross or Victoria Station in London, and these large hubs were connected to many smaller hubs. Hubs correlated with the children's learning profiles, meaning larger, well-connected hubs seen in the brain were a good indicator of the areas where the children showed strong abilities and poorly connected hubs within the brain indicated perceived challenge areas within their learning profiles.

As discussed, learning is always a sensory business. It stands to reason that sensory signals travelling into the brain as electrical impulses from a child's most useful senses would feed into specific areas of the brain associated with that sense. Hence, the more signals coming into specific areas, the more connectivity there would be in that area, creating larger hubs. Equally, in senses (or elements within senses), where a child struggles with sensory access, less information would flow through to the brain, creating smaller hubs in those areas.

Hubs which connected across sensory brain regions were also observed. Interestingly, synesthetes (people who experience synaesthesia) have been observed to have more connections between the parts of the brain that control their senses. This means that areas receiving less sensory information may connect to other, more highly-connected areas, to process sensory information.

The organisation of hubs could be the neurological representation of sensory abundance and pattern recognition. Although autistic sensory profiles differ from person to person, this type of connectivity could underlie many traits seen across autistic individuals. When a child is accessing lots of sensory information, this could present in the brain as a busy hub that is processing and storing a huge amount of information (underlying monotropism). It is easy to imagine that the areas with more connections will be extremely active with electro-chemical activity. These hubs may become easily overloaded. Just as with any overloaded circuit, hubs can 'blow a fuse' or stop working. The next logical step is clear: children with sensory abundance and busy brain hubs are much more likely to experience sensory overload and shutdown. These hubs can be overloaded by too much information: this might happen in an environment with excessive sensory stimulation or when a child has to process lots of challenging sensory information, such as taking in lots of spoken instructions (especially if spoken language is not easy for them to access).

Autistic children who focus on their sensory surroundings more than most may also become extremely vigilant around possible sensory triggers. Autistic children are often much more connected to sensory aspects in their environment; even small changes can be unnerving. For many autistic children, changing their environment can create anxiety and confusion because it goes against their current conceptual understanding. When that autistic child is minimally- or non-speaking, such a change can be incredibly difficult. To better understand this experience, imagine that every time you left your house, you noticed that the houses on your street were changing and that each day, more and more slates and bricks were removed. Each day, you notice more and more change. By day five, you come out, and all the houses have disappeared. This would be unnerving.

Now, imagine your neurosensory profile means you cannot communicate, so you cannot ask anyone what is happening. Consider how many questions you would have and how much anxiety that could trigger.

Although the above example may sound extreme, Chris Packham, an autistic television personality, explains that this is exactly how he experiences environments. He explains that when he goes into a forest he walks in regularly, he notices one branch out of place. This change means he needs to completely reconfigure how he has visually recorded that environment in his head. This gives a glimpse into how confusing environmental changes can be for some autistic children.

Having hubs of activity in areas of the brain that are not expected alters the way autistic children respond to and interact with everything around them. Autistic children have been tasked with the impossible. They have been asked to override their own autonomy over their environment, their interactions and their responses (which would fulfil their natural 'ways of being') and have been told instead to act, interact and endure in places completely set up for non-autistic children. This leads to traits currently framed as 'autistic deficits' and 'challenging behaviours' when, in reality, they are naturally occurring responses to situations not of their making.

PART SIX:

AUTISTIC COMMUNICATION AND PLAY

'When a flower doesn't bloom, you fix the environment in which it grows, not the flower.'

Alexander Den Heijer

When autistic children try to integrate into social settings, there are often many barriers to accessing speaking, listening and learning in typical environments. Alongside this, autistic internal processes give rise to either necessary or inevitable traits when attempting to live in a world that is not structured around their requirements.

Autistic neurosensory profiles mean that autistic children experience the world fundamentally differently from many of their peers. This difference can give rise to challenges when autistic and non-autistic children interact socially. The onus is currently often placed on autistic children to integrate and adapt their own communication and play. The next few sections highlight why this is an unfair expectation and discuss how more social support could facilitate better autistic social relationships.

The goal should be to ensure that autistic children no longer have to navigate inherently challenging social settings and situations.

Communication divergence and autistic languages

Now we understand that autistic children's primary mode of information gathering from sensory inputs can be different from that of most children. We now move from considering sensory input to focusing on sensory output. A child who is accessing divergent sensory patterns may be unable to tune into spoken communication in an expected way or at an expected age. As discussed in the pattern recognition chapter, they will still access information and seek connection through communication, but this communication may manifest as a first language other than speech. Autistic children who pick up on the written code may become hyperlexic (early readers), primarily picking up their information from books. If and when these children start to speak, they may do so in an unexpected way. Some might predominantly pick up the pictorial code, leading them to think in pictures, and if and when they start to speak, it may be based on their pictorial understanding of the world. Whatever an autistic child's first language, their communication journey may look very different from that of their non-autistic peers.

So, how do autistic children build their first languages? Speech is not necessarily the first type of communication an autistic child accesses, although they may hear voices. Some autistic babies and children might listen to voices as an almost musical experience where the pitch of voices is of interest to them, or like Donna Williams, the autistic author, they may hear words as a mumble jumble. Alternatively, a child might pick up on the poetic pattern of rhyming words.

There are many ways a child might hear 'words' before they acquire conventional meaning. The meaning of words is built through contextualising those words in interactions and environments. Long before children start speaking, they build up this contextual understanding. When my nephew, Jay, was starting to copy speech around age two we would visit the duck pond daily, and I would point to the ducks and say 'duck'. After a while, he repeated this, pointing and saying 'duck, duck, duck'. He then started pointing at anything with wings, shouting 'duck'. He had learned that all the things that looked like a bird with wings might be called a duck; his brain had made a prediction and tested the theory.

'Not quite,' I explained, pointing at the birds in the

trees. 'Bird.' After a few weeks of showing him this differentiation, Jay went back to the ducks and shouted 'duck' and then pointed at the birds in the trees and shouted 'bird'. In this way, he was building his contextual understanding through his environment and social interactions.

But before the above process can occur, children need to *hear* the separate words as just that... *separate words*. Explaining a word in context can be helpful, but what if the child you are explaining to cannot hear the words you are saying or cannot see the things you are pointing to? For a child experiencing sensorily busy environments, where the visual and auditory input is all flowing into their brain, the words and context may simply blend into all the other noises and visual stimuli in the environment. Children who experience synaesthesia might see colours and symbols floating in the air instead of hearing specific words and tying these to the 'duck' you are pointing to. Pointing becomes meaningless when the child has no idea what you are pointing at within all that visual busyness, and words might be just another sound within the cacophony of sounds.

We must distinguish between autistic children with verbal apraxia and NSD autistic children. This is because autistic children with verbal apraxia may be receiving sensory input from spoken words, but their motor abilities might prevent them from expressing that knowledge. Although they may present similar traits to NSD autistic children, this difference means that they are not experiencing the world exactly as NSD autistic children do. Children with verbal apraxia sometimes express meaningless words and phrases that do not convey their underlying knowledge; they state that these can feel like uncontrollable tics. These children may benefit from motor support alongside finding a communication system that works best for them. If and when these children have access to a useful communication system, people are often astounded by their inner knowledge. However, this should not come as a surprise, as an inability to speak has no bearing on cognitive ability.

In the case of NSD autistic children, their brains and their senses will be busy looking for meaningful communication and environmental patterns that they *can* plug into. The interesting thing with Jay is that he did not seem to build his speech or his contextual understanding predominantly through spoken communication. Long before speaking in full sentences, he would copy words and phrases as we read to him. Very early on, around the age of two, he would pick up a book he knew well and mimic all the words. The way the words sounded was not always clear, but it sounded similar to the words in the book. Because he was so young, we assumed that he was simply copying the sounds. We now know that he was probably picking up on the written code and using spoken cues as a secondary way of accessing and using communication.

Here, Heidi, an autistic adult, reflects on her childhood experiences of accessing the visual, written code as her 'first language':

The way I would receive information. It would be visual if it were written up on the board. Much of it would be from what was written down or from reading or just thinking about the material in front of me ... [learning] was very mildly supplemented by listening.

It appears to be the case (at least for some children) that the less sensorily busy an environment, the more accessible spoken communication can be, especially when we consider the conference effect. Usually, in a child's early years, they are read to at night, in a low arousal environment, with the curtains drawn, when the world outside is quieter, and the sounds in the house such as vacuum cleaners and washing machines are mostly turned off. For neurosensory divergent children, this sort of environment might make accessing spoken words easier, especially when accompanied by a visual cue. For children like Jay, who could access the written code (reading), this environment might enable them to relate the sounds they hear to the letters and words they see. In this way, memories and prior learning begin to build around memorising this written code (as opposed to primarily embedding the spoken code). This might happen early (hyperlexia), or written letters may be something the child uses to scaffold their access to communication later in their communication journey. Not using speech as a first language does not mean that all autistic children are non-speaking. Many may be highly verbal, but their communication style is likely to diverge if they are accessing communication divergently from non-autistic children.

For Jay, it became obvious that it was books, alphabet flashcards, number flashcards and all different kinds of written codes that he was plugging into. This meant he had a consistent way of accessing communication, which he would supplement through the spoken words he *could* access. I imagine these spoken words were accessed sporadically. He certainly homed in on the words which were meaningful to him. We now know that Jay was building an almost photographic memory of written words; he had (and still has) a Filofax of words in his brain, which he could recall quickly. He also memorised phrases and began applying these in the appropriate context.

It was becoming apparent that Jay's communication was building in an unusual way. I have since learned that this is known as a Gestalt way of learning language. Most children have some form of gestalt language where phrases or chunks of words are applied to specific contexts. Gestalt phrases a child might use include 'What's that?' or 'Going out now'. These are mini scripts that the child memorises and puts together in meaning-making. However, these gestalt scripts do not always describe exactly what the child is trying to say. In the case of Jay, he had learned (from books and TV shows) that 'I am Thomas' is what Thomas the Tank Engine says when he is introducing himself, so Jay would run up to other children and say 'I am Thomas' as this seemed to fit contextually for him. Similarly, a child might say, 'Are you okay?' when they have hurt themselves because they hear other people use this phrase when they are hurt.

This type of communication is often called echolalia, where a child repeats what they have heard. Echolalia is common in most toddlers, but because autistic children often use this skill later in their communication journey and may use it for longer, it is often thought of as an abnormal autistic trait.

Gestalt language building adds a layer of complication to language acquisition. Autistic children who learn this way will be marrying speech to their dominant way of information gathering. For example, a visual learner who has plugged into environmental visual patterns (such as how a shadow falls on a tree or the composition of a scene) has to go through their mental Filofax of images to make sense of the spoken words they are hearing. For children who have built their language this way, listening to purely spoken words may be tiring, as they are continually translating the words into their own 'first language' to meaning-make.

Jules, an autistic adult, explains how she built her knowledge of the world, stating that her speech was not always reliable. Instead, her visual memories were her stored sense-making process:

I've got a very strong visual memory. I can go back in time like watching a film of each year of my life, and I don't remember words very well, but the visual is all there; it's almost like playing a tape.

Jules was not storing written letters like Jay. Instead, she was storing images. Jules remembers finding early communication incredibly challenging. She would quietly observe other children and play alongside them.

I had no idea how to speak to other children; it felt like I was from a different planet. I preferred to be in my own imaginary world. It always felt like it was such a huge effort to attempt to join in with other children talking.

Not only do autistic children need to access, embed and translate spoken instructions and expectations into their 'first language', they also have to act on those instructions. This would undoubtedly impact many processes associated with executive functioning. It is not a straightforward case of accessing words and then responding.

Dom, an autistic adult, reflects on the fact that he thinks mainly in written words and how this has impacted his thought processes:

When I think about anything in my mind, it is always in writing; I see what people say in a written form in my head and then have to translate it back to speech so I can say what I want to say. It is an unconscious process now, but I imagine it wasn't as a child.

Millie is diagnosed ADHD/ autistic. She *did* pick up spoken words early but explains that she does not think in words, pictures *or* graphemes (written words) but instead connects through whole-body emotions.

'With me, it is like no specific sense is in charge with either my communication or my thought process. I seem to use all my senses at once. I can be pulled towards whichever things pique my interest. I have to connect emotionally to things to learn and I do not always connect or remember spoken words. When I was little, I also didn't always pick up on visual social cues, but now I do. It is like I feel their emotion. It can be draining to experience so keenly the emotions and judgement of others.'

TJ, an autistic writer with unreliable speech, shares that she can visualise the words she intends to express in her mind, yet when it comes to articulating the sentence, unintended words often intrude into her speech. This makes it difficult to depend on her own translation process[71].

As is the case for these autistic adults, autistic children's communication process is not as straightforward as translating a spoken language such as French to English. Autistic children have to context-make in a non-speech-based language and then translate this into spoken words; this is a highly complex process. When an autistic child begins to communicate with single words, gestalt scripts and pauses, it might sound stilted and clunky. This is often misconstrued as a lack of ability. In reality,

71 www.instagram.com. (TJ.). Instagram. [online] Available at: https://www.instagram.com/reel/CwTKEEfMwDY/?utm_source=ig_web_copy_link&igshid=MzRlODBiNWFlZA== [Accessed 26 Aug. 2023].

having to translate, script and context-make causes speech to be less intuitive for autistic children. This is often described as autistic children having problems with information processing, executive functioning and social communication issues, but I would counter this. I would say they are experiencing barriers to accessing the way that information is being relayed and the way they are expected to respond (i.e. in spoken words).

The late Mel Baggs (whose pronouns are they/them), who was an autistic non-speaking advocate and blogger, described their own experience as being in constant communication with their environment.[72] They pointed out that autistic people are expected to learn spoken communication but that the rest of society often fails to learn autistic communication. Autistic, non-speech based communication is often equated with a lack of ability, but their brains tell a different story with hyperconnected areas in unexpected parts of the brain. It is probable that accessing spoken communication as a second language has the same impact on autistic brains as bilingualism, where there is more connectivity in unexpected areas of the brain. Even when an autistic child is not using speech, if they are accessing and using multiple types of sensory input (such as visual and tactile) to build concepts, this too could present as multiple languages. Bilingual children are recorded as having larger brain sizes, as are autistic children. It is probable that switching between languages and in-brain

72   silentmiaow (2007). In My Language. YouTube. Available at: https://www.youtube.com/watch?v=JnylM1hI2jc.

translation presents as divergent brain connectivity compared to single-language speakers.

A child's first language will likely be built around their pattern recognition. For a child who is primarily accessing the tactile (who learns by touching and feeling the world around them), their communication journey will look significantly different from that of a child mainly accessing visual codes and patterns (who thinks and learns through images) and different again from a child who initially visually picks up the written word and grammatical codes (who thinks in written words). It is important to acknowledge that any autistic child, whether pre-speaking, non-speaking or speaking, has to put a lot of effort into communicating with a predominantly speaking world.

There is often a lack of aligned communication between autistic and non-autistic children, which often acts as a barrier. Autistic children tend to communicate more literally because spoken language is effortful for them, so they use it to... do what it says on the tin. For autistic children, spoken language is a means to communicate what is inside their heads! The issue comes when autistic children attempt to interact with non-autistic children. Often, when autistic children attempt to use their non-intuitive second language (speech) to communicate, they may enter conversations in unusual ways, jumping in or saying something that does not fit with the conversation. Non-autistic children may already be proficient in speaking, listening and back-and-forth conversations. Many autistic adults reflect on this period of their childhood as confusing, and nearly all the autistic adults and children I know have experienced rejection for their own style of communication.

Autistic children may not be as involved in social back-and-forth conversations, both due to their sensory access and because of failed attempts to join such conversations. Instead, they must find innovative ways to learn social communication; many do this through TV programmes. When Jay turned six, he found subtitles on the television and has never looked back. He told me how much it helped him. He said tuning into the words without the written subtitles was much more complicated. He is not the only one. Many autistic people use subtitles or visuals to aid their access to speech. This is also one reason gaming can be such a positive experience for autistic children and young people. The demands of speaking and listening are significantly reduced while allowing them to access the social aspect of playing a game with friends. Although it may not be suitable for all autistic children, screen time is positive for many.

Sensory access and missing expected knowledge

If autistic children are unable to easily access and join in with social conversations, how does this impact their social journey and conceptual knowledge? This is currently framed as them having social and emotional deficits, issues with reciprocal conversations and empathy, and a tendency to isolate themselves. I would counter this and state that autistic children are trying desperately to access and connect with the social world but that it is the social world that presents barriers to that connection.

When Jay was young, I used to occasionally go to the local playgroup with him and his Mum. There Jay would happily parallel play near other children, he would find trains to carry around, and if there were a Thomas the Tank, he would be in seventh heaven! But when he reached the age of two and the children around him started to have early conversations, we noticed a striking difference. I remember Jay just staring at the other children chatting away with each other. He looked utterly bemused by the chatter around him and sat quietly, playing with his trains and observing the confusing scene. It seemed like Jay was entirely used to the adults around him chatting, but now his peers were doing it, and he couldn't fathom it.

One day, when his mother picked him up from Nursery, his very lovely nursery teacher asked if Jay had always been mute! As I worked in the nursery, I could discuss this at length with his teacher and explain that he wasn't mute and was already reading. The teacher looked amazed and seemed unconvinced. It struck me that Jay was presenting as mute in a noisy nursery environment but was talking in his home, where it was quieter. I asked her to take him somewhere quiet with a book, and sure enough, he read to her. It appeared to be the noisy environment that was altering Jay's communication journey. While Jay's peers were having reciprocal conversations and learning from one another, Jay was learning from books and building gestalt language. He would happily interact with other minimally speaking children, taking part in running and chasing games.

This probably meant that ideas usually embedded through reciprocal conversations weren't being fed to Jay. Even during story time in the nursery, if he could not see the written text, I imagine his teacher's words would mostly float away into the many other noises he could hear. Concepts about the seasons, about sharing, about safety, about wiggly worms – so many concepts taught through spoken interactions were just floating away. Jay accessed only intermittently information usually passed on through reciprocal conversations and speech-based teaching. This sporadic access to communication is likely to have altered Jay's conceptual learning journey. Many autistic children may be hearing far fewer words than their similarly aged peers and, therefore, building less of their conceptual knowledge around speech. This means autistic children are often filling in the blanks to create their own understanding of the world.

To illustrate this, let's draw a comparison with dyslexic children's experience of reading. Imagine a passage with certain parts redacted. This is how many dyslexic children access pieces of writing, making it challenging to grasp the full meaning. Dyslexic children often rely on clues and prior knowledge to fill in the missing information. This barrier makes it hugely challenging for dyslexic children to keep up with their similarly-aged peers. Imagine these missing conceptual learnings occurring within the spoken code. Moreover, consider that an autistic child may face a double access issue when they have divergent access in multiple senses. In such cases, they might miss words and struggle to interpret body language and visual cues.

It is clear to see that autistic children need support with access to communication, whether this is speech or another form of communication. Jay's parents were lucky enough to find a communication support that worked for Jay in the form of Lego therapy. These are sessions where children take turns to create a Lego model. Throughout these interactions, there is a teacher who acts as a facilitator, a child who finds the Lego block, an engineer who says where it should go and a builder who puts the block onto the model. This was always conducted in a quiet room with set rules to follow, a structure and written activity cards to aid spoken communication. Although this helped Jay build confidence, it would not be right for every autistic child. Each autistic child will need their own set of supports based on their own first language and sensory profile, but finding strategies to aid their autistic communication is of paramount importance.

Communication and autistic interests

Autistic children who are not as focused on spoken communication might instead become adept at enjoying the things their sensory profile *does* home in on. This means they often begin to focus intensely on the things they enjoy. There are fewer outside influences from the spoken and social world around them, which means they can revel in their interests. In this way, autistic brains are steered towards specialising in subjects and interests based on their individual pattern spotting. This type of specialising presents externally as monotropic traits (such as having highly focused interests) and internally as brain connectivity that diverges from the expected.

Communication builds around the words, images or concepts that children access most often and the things that are most meaningful to them. During these hyper-focused moments, a child might seem unreachable and wholly absorbed in their own world. This skill is particularly valuable for children with neurosensory abundance as it allows them to focus their attention, helping them cope better with their environment. Autistic individuals often describe this experience as highly enjoyable and all-encompassing.

Reflecting on her childhood, Heidi, an autistic adult, remembers being fully immersed in these moments of focused engagement:

I enjoyed being in my own head, and I was always writing stories and writing songs and just being interested in everything. I was so busy being interested in everything.

Here, Jules, an autistic adult, states that she gets lots of enjoyment out of just getting lost in her own thoughts:

I wouldn't change my brain because my brain is almost like an entertainment system. ... I can go into my brain, and I have so many thoughts that I find fascinating about the world. It's almost like my own documentary; I've never been able to put this into words; it's really hard as a neurodiverse person, isn't it, to explain what goes on in your brain. In a way, it's a gift to have those skills, even though you lack other skills.

Yet, this can sometimes be frustrating for the people around autistic children. Dom, an autistic adult, told me what it is like to be pulled into a 'focus tunnel'.

Often when a TV is on, or any screen, my focus is pulled into the screen. It looks like I am not listening or distracted to those around me, but it can help me focus on what people are saying.

Leah, an autistic child, explains that sometimes she can become so engrossed in an activity that her mind becomes really busy and the activity is all she can focus on.

I can hardly hear my Mum calling me because I am so engaged in whatever activity I am doing. My Mum can find it frustrating and says it feels like I am ignoring her, but really, I am just very focused.

Most people can easily switch their attention between tasks, but switching attention in a monotropic mind can be more challenging. Leah told me it feels like meditation, where the outside world melts away. Trying to bring her thoughts back into the 'real world' can take time. The theory of monotropism is a far cry from the historical framing of autistic people as withdrawn, delayed, or disordered. Instead, it builds an understanding that autistic children may be learning divergently and possess abilities to hyperfocus on things that fall outside of the norm.

In certain autistic children, this focused style of attention, combined with their ability to spot divergent patterns, can give rise to what I refer to as 'subject think'. The term 'subject think' encapsulates the intensity and enthusiasm with which these children immerse themselves in their favourite topics. It highlights the remarkable capacity of autistic individuals to delve deeply into areas of fascination. Sharing their passion and knowledge about their interests becomes a significant way for autistic children to seek connection with others. This is often called info dumping. Info dumping can lead to a disconnect between the way autistic and non-autistic children communicate.

'Groupthink', 'subject think' and conformity

In psychology, the social identity approach of 'groupthink' focuses on the process by which groups make distinctions on who is to be included and who is to be excluded. These interactions can inform private understandings of oneself because individual members base their own understanding of self on how they are perceived within a group. For the purposes of this book, I am interested in the subtle ways groupthink materialises throughout early development and how it becomes a staple of daily life for the majority of children. This is the type of thinking that evolves when children form into cohesive groups.

There are often hierarchies within social groups, and this happens even with very young children. In group settings, non-autistic children often engage in social pattern recognition, closely observing their peers' reactions, including both their spoken language and non-verbal cues, to assess the group members' emotions. As a result, some children may start to follow their peers' lead. Some children may adapt to seek acceptance by being friendly and non-confrontational, while others who are more assertive might navigate the delicate balance of taking a leadership role within the group while also consistently seeking approval from their peers to maintain group support. Non-autistic children have differing degrees of success assimilating and fitting into group dynamics, but as I will explain, autistic children are naturally developing along their own pathway and 'groupthink' may not feature as a natural part of their development. That is not to say they cannot be part of a group, but they may find group conformity at odds with their natural ways of being.

Autistic memory also plays a part in this process. Memory is how the brain encodes, stores, and retrieves information when needed. In autistic children, the information most accessible will be easiest to encode and store. Conceptual understanding and memories build into brain connectivity, meaning autistic children will have large areas of stored information around their first languages. In many autistic children, this will not be predominantly speech. This is an important distinction between autistic memory and non-autistic memory. Many non-autistic children can hold a spoken thought in their memory while simultaneously listening to the conversation. When they feel it appropriate, they can add their little memorised nugget of wisdom into that conversation. It is entirely different for many autistic children. They can instantly forget spoken thoughts or face challenges translating these thoughts quickly enough, especially when simultaneously trying to follow spoken conversations. This probably underlies the autistic tendency to jump in rather than wait patiently in a conversation. Some autistic children are also less adept at remembering faces and facial expressions. Meaning they are less able to read and decode their peers' reactions. This, combined with subject think and info dumping in which they monologue about their interests, can cause a disconnect between non-autistic and autistic children. This can lead to autistic children being socially rejected.

Many autistic children do not take part in the process of assimilating into groups as early as their peers (if at all). Or, if they are joining groups, their focus is less on the group dynamics and more on seeking connection through their interests. Autistic children have told me that integrating into social groups in expected ways is an impossible task. For a Gestalt learner of language, following a dynamic spoken conversation is in itself effortful, and this is added to the fact that many conversations happen in sensorially busy playgrounds. So, while autistic children are focusing on the mechanics of following and taking part in a conversation, they also have to form their own concepts, translate these from their first language and then feed their ideas into the conversation at the correct point while simultaneously following the evolving conversation. As you can imagine, sustaining this level of focus to take part in fast-paced reciprocal conversations is exhausting.

Instead, natural autistic communication often involves more monologue to monologue (or info dumping). The feeling of getting everything out that they want to say in one big flow takes away the mental load of reciprocal conversations. Some autistic children are more comfortable taking part in reciprocal conversations on a familiar subject. However, attempting to assimilate into group conversations based around social interactions and norms can be effortful.

In many ways, autistic children have more autonomy over their own interests and beliefs because they are not being moulded by 'groupthink'. Connection for lots of autistic children is interest or subject-driven, meaning they will make social connections using the things they love and feel most comfortable with. Autistic children are often so excited by their interests that they assume others will share their excitement. As I will cover in empathy, sharing similar experiences is often autistic children's love language. However, this difference in communication style can lead to misunderstandings.

Autistic children may communicate in a more literal and less socially complex way. That is not to say they lack complexity of thought – only complexity of expected thought. At the point when group dynamics become more complex and unwritten social rules further develop, autistic children are often confused about how they are 'supposed' to access and sustain social connections within these rules. Alongside this, autistic interests and speech may not appear 'age-appropriate'. Communication differences can mean that some autistic children appear younger with slower speech, and others may appear older with much more formal speech. A huge amount of unconscious communication bias impacts autistic children and their families, whereby their communication is marked out as odd. It is worth mentioning that many autistic children grow up in neurodivergent families with other people who are also subject thinkers and info dumpers (because neurodivergence is highly heritable). They, too, may have experienced the pain of being excluded or judged for the way they communicated (too much, too little or in unexpected ways). Communication bias plays a big part in identity rejection and autistic trauma.

I also want to discuss small talk, as this is another part of conversation that autistic subject thinkers view as confusing. Think back to the beginning of this book. Did I start by asking about the weather? Or what TV shows you currently watch? No, I went straight in, talking about this book being a fight song. This got me thinking: we don't use small talk in any other context of imparting information, not in books, not in TV, not in films. So, what is the psychology behind small talk? Small talk is the use of unimportant and uncontroversial matters to avoid feeling awkward or vulnerable. The use of small talk assumes that when one enters into a conversation, you are vulnerable because conversations can be unsafe situations where people judge and exclude. So, small talk becomes a way of not oversharing or not sharing personal details. It is also used at the beginning of conversations and may become deeper once both people feel comfortable sharing. When autistic children first leap into communicating through joyfully sharing their interests, they are not expecting to be met with judgement. There will be some children who, due to divergent visual sensory access, may not even register that judgement on faces and others who, over time, feel overwhelmed by the amount of judgement and exclusion they receive, simply for communicating in a natural way for them.

Communication bias and groupthink are rooted in the idea that social conformity and communication uniformity are expected and this is policed by both children and adults. Current research around autistic socialising often positions autistic children as the ones who socially isolate themselves. But as I have laid out, many autistic children who access communication divergently are excluded by those around them as opposed to isolating themselves. This means that if and when they try to assimilate with their similarly aged peers, their journey is often fraught with confusion. Groups who do not understand or accept autistic profiles may not accept them socially and may actively reject autistic traits.

Autistic children can find acceptance in groups of children with similar interests and communication styles (often other neurodivergent children). This is not to say all autistic children get on: they do not! However, children with similar neurosensory profiles may well get along in a group dynamic. This means that in an average mainstream school, there will be far fewer opportunities for autistic children to build strong, authentic connections and find acceptance. When finding a genuine connection is not possible, autistic children may feel safer staying on the periphery of groups, become increasingly isolated, or resort to masking, attempting to conform to groupthink and non-autistic communication styles.

Autistic children are often not scaffolded in their own communication style. A good comparison for this is that if there were a deaf child in a mainstream school who could only sign to communicate, they might struggle to connect to their peers and feel very isolated. Their peers might try to learn some sign language to communicate, but that deeper connection may be limited, and they would likely miss out on lots of the social aspects of school. In fact, in some mainstream schools, deaf teachers have been brought in to support the whole school in learning sign language to create a connection between deaf and hearing children. When autistic children struggle to communicate with their non-autistic peers, both sides are often left confused and fail to forge close connections.

I was recently talking to a young non-autistic adult reflecting on her childhood; she explained that she knew how to accept autistic children because she had been in classes with autistic children. However, she mentioned that as these autistic children got older, one autistic child in particular continued to greet everyone with, 'What is your name?' She said this became annoying by the time they were thirteen or fourteen years old, and the non-autistic children would say, 'You know my name; stop asking.' When I explained that this was probably an echolalic script that the autistic child probably used as a greeting rather than having forgotten their names, she said she had never considered this a possibility. Knowing this made her reassess her classmates' responses, and she stated that had they known this, they might have responded more patiently.

Autistic children who do not use speech as their first

language still seek those deep connections, which are often easier within neurodivergent communities. Just as with deaf and blind children, the presence of shared experiences, interests, communication styles, and humour can lead to cultural differences between individuals who are autistic and those who are not. Exploring and providing additional research and support is imperative to understand this disconnect.

I need to state that even though communication is a spectrum, where some autistic children may be proficient speakers, they may still struggle with the complexity and layers of social norms and reciprocal conversations. Equally, some autistic children cannot speak or are unreliable speakers, but that does not mean they cannot communicate or understand what the people around them are saying. Tiffany Hammond, an autistic writer, has written a children's book called *A Day with No Words*[73] that highlights the isolation and judgement that non-speaking autistic children can face on a daily basis. In it, her son is judged by others simply for stimming in a way that calms and soothes him.

Due to sensory access challenges, divergent pattern recognition, divergent first languages, monotropic thinking, missing speech-based conceptual knowledge, and interest-driven learning styles, the early years of an autistic child's life differ significantly from those of a non-autistic child. It is no wonder that autistic adults

---

73   Hammond, T. (2023). A Day With No Words. Wheat Penny Press.

often say they felt like aliens when they reflect on their childhood. Alis Rowe, an autistic advocate, explains this in her glass jar theory[74], stating that autistic children often feel on the outside of social groups, staying on the periphery as if they are stuck in a glass jar, unable to break through social barriers.

Autistic communication lived-experience

Communicating as a subject thinker in a world full of groupthinkers can be like talking to people who speak another language. Initial attempts to bridge this gap can lead to issues. I remember watching Jay just walk up to a group of children, no introduction, no pre-amble, straight in with, 'I have a fantastic operating system on my computer at home. What do you have?' The children he was attempting to connect with looked perplexed; a few giggled while Jay waited expectantly for an answer. The other children had no idea how to respond, and both Jay and the other children failed to make any sort of meaningful connection through their interaction. For autistic children, often their whole life up until they enter the social sphere has been about finding joy by focusing on their interests; sharing that joy is what motivates them socially. However, their efforts to connect are often rejected and can lead to bullying and ridicule (see identity rejection).

---

74   The Girl with the Curly Hair. (n.d.). The Glass Jar Theory. [online] Available at: https://thegirlwiththecurlyhair.co.uk/animat ed-film/the-glass-jar-theory/ [Accessed 14 Aug. 2023].

Jules is an autistic adult, and she remembers feeling like her style of communication was not appealing to other children:

[I had] this issue of not knowing how to talk to kids and just standing there being really awkward or monologuing at them. I do remember that up to about Year Three, I didn't really have any friends. I played alongside children, not talking. ...so I was quite lonely because I guess I didn't know how to enter the friendship groups of other girls.

Jules remembers struggling to communicate because, as she put it,

I communicate verbally in a much simpler way than most people. Nowadays, I prefer to write than talk because I have time to think things through.

Conversely, Heidi, another autistic adult, says that her style of communication was less accepted by her peers because of her advanced language and word choices.

I learned to read when I was three, like the tail end of three. I was self-taught.

I was just kind of pedantic; I'd use big words, and everyone thought I was posh because I would use fancy words. My mum said I spoke like an adult – I was like a mini adult from very young. I don't know the age, but I was hyperverbal and would just come out with these long, sophisticated sentences.

Heidi explained that other children teased her for her word choices and that she even got labelled as arrogant by her peers and her teachers due to the way she spoke.

[When I talked about my academic abilities], it would look like arrogance, but it did feel pretty factual. I wasn't sat there thinking I'm better than you... my self-esteem wasn't very good, I don't think - I always felt like, ooh, you know, you probably don't like me.

Both Jules and Heidi remember finding it very difficult to fit into social groups, often only finding a select few friends whom they could get on with. Many autistic children feel this social rejection keenly, and many autistic adults have reflected on the trauma this caused them. Damien Milton discusses this disconnect in terms of autistic people having their own culture and communication. It is often the case that when neurodivergent children find one another, they can create good bonds because of their shared culture. However, there are fewer of their cultural buddies in any one playground, so creating opportunities for these types of groupings is important. Identity rejection is extremely damaging to autistic children and young people, and steps should be taken to create safe and accepting spaces; this includes teaching whole communities how to act inclusively.

Non- and pre-speaking autistic communication

Non-speaking or pre-speaking autistic children experience many barriers when attempting to communicate with a predominantly speaking world. They often have to use their bodies to communicate their wants, needs and their distress. Body communication is often heavily judged, yet for some non-speaking or pre-speaking autistic children, it is their primary means of communication. Even some speaking autistic children resort to body communication at times. When children express their emotions through actions rather than words, it can sometimes lead to judgement from others. For example, a non-speaking child who is overwhelmed when crowded by other children cannot tell anyone. They have to show their discomfort by pushing the other children away.

Non-autistic people often struggle to understand sensory experiences that overwhelm autistic children. This puts non-speaking and pre-speaking autistic children in a vulnerable position as they may be unable to effectively communicate their distress. When these children use body communication to express their opposition to something, it may be misunderstood as defiance or bad behaviour when, in reality, it could be their only way of seeking autonomy over having their basic needs met.

Some speech therapist advocate for redirection when a child uses body communication to express themselves. However, this is not always optimal for autistic children. In a world built around speech, having their only form of communication ignored or redirected can be isolating. Before Jay became fluent in speech, his Mum received advice from a therapist to promote speech-based communication and discourage body communication. When Jay tried to express his needs by leading them to items or through gesturing, they were encouraged to guide him to ask for things using words instead. However, this approach confused Jay and other methods like pictures and signing didn't work either. Jay became frustrated at times, and his parents eventually decided to follow Jay's lead and simply named the item when he led them to it. This sparked meaningful interactions where Jay eventually combined his body communication with spoken words.

Augmentative and Alternative Communication (AAC)

Many autistic children benefit from accessing and using communication other than speech. Augmentative and alternative communication (AAC) includes communication devices, systems, strategies and/ or tools that replace or support speech.[75] When considering a communication system for autistic children, parents often face a limited range of options. Many children are initially offered speech and language training, where children learn to use spoken words. When speech and language support does not lead to meaningful communication, autistic children might be offered Makaton[76] (a unique signing language that combines signs, symbols, and speech) or picture-based systems[77], where children use pictures instead of words (for instance, using a picture of a school instead of saying 'school'). Nowadays, picture-based systems are available on electronic devices.[78] This allows children

---

75   www.assistiveware.com. (n.d.). What is AAC? - AssistiveWare. [online] Available at: https://www.assistiveware.com/learn-aac/ what-is-aac#:~:text=AAC%20is%20short%20for%20Augmentative.

76   (n.d.). Available at: https://files.eric.ed.gov/fulltext/ED291193. pdf.

77   Bondy, A. and Frost, L. (2017). Picture Exchange Communication System (PECS)® |. [online] Pyramid Educational Consultants UK. Available at: https://pecs-unitedkingdom.com/pecs/.

78   AssistiveWare (2019). Proloquo2Go - AAC app with symbols - AssistiveWare. [online] Assistiveware.com. Available at: https://www. assistiveware.com/products/proloquo2go.

to select a picture, triggering a voice which relays the child's intended message.

While these communication methods have proven successful with many autistic children, they may not be suitable for every child due to each child's sensory profile and first language. For instance, Jay did not respond well to visual aids or sign language. If his parents had continued to insist on using these methods, it might have delayed his progress in communication through written and spoken words.

The limited number of communication systems offered to autistic children can leave those who require different approaches feeling lost. Mirenda,[79] an educational researcher, states that unconventional communication options should always be considered. She believes that limited options are offered due to assumptions made about autistic individuals and that new ways to support autistic communication should be invented. It is often the case that parents do find their own unconventional methods. One such example is the use of letterboards, where a child is shown letters on a board and points to them to form words. Though not widely recognised, many children and parents credit this system with enabling communication.

Although a small minority of autistic children may have learning difficulties when it comes to communication,

79   Mirenda, P. (2008). A Back Door Approach to Autism and AAC. Augmentative and Alternative Communication, 24(3), pp.220–234. doi:https://doi.org/10.1080/08990220802388263.

it is also useful to consider whether some autistic children may be experiencing challenges associated with accessibility. Mapping a child's Neurosensory profile could be instrumental in finding the right communication support. For instance, children who gather information primarily through touch might benefit from a tactile communication system similar to braille. A child who connects emotionally to music might thrive using songs or letters on a musical keyboard. Children who enjoy replaying video clips could use these as a form of communication, and those who use body communication might benefit from a universal body communication system.

Speech and Language support can be very helpful, but autistic children may need to develop different first languages in order to access further second languages (such as speech). It should also be mentioned that speech is not always the goal; finding a communication tool that is meaningful for the autistic child is the goal. When a useful tool is found, it can be very helpful if the people around that child model and use the same tool. Similar to acquiring any language, immersive learning is more effective than attempting to learn a language in isolation.

Exploratory Play

Both speech and non-speech based communication can be an important part of play. Throughout 'expected' play, children develop their speech as they recount spoken conversations and narratives around their play. Autistic children's play may look quite different from this. Jay's play was quite investigative. He loved Thomas the Tank Engine. He copied phrases from the Thomas shows he had watched, pushing the trains from one station to the next. Jay's lack of spoken narrative and his style of play might have been traditionally framed as a lack of imagination, but Jay did not lack imagination. In fact, he would often fall into peals of laughter or smile at something only he could see in his own mind. It was just that Jay wasn't able to express this reliably through speech. Through traditional autism framing, Jay would also have been described as having restricted interests, but to us, he was just delighting in his interests, which sparked *such* joy; how could one call that restricted?

Jay's parents fully embraced each new interest, which could last for years or come and go in a few months. They went on every train going with him and would travel for miles to Thomas Land, and he would beam from ear to ear every single time. After trains, Jay became interested in lifts; his parents spent hours on lifts with him, pressing buttons and enjoying going up and down in different lifts. Some people worried about Jay's strange interests, but his parents never wavered in fulfilling their child's wishes to try different lifts everywhere they visited. Next, Jay discovered traffic lights and enjoyed playing with his toy traffic lights at home, watching them follow a sequence. At every turn, professionals advised Jay's parents to encourage him to play with the toys other children his age were playing with. The professionals voiced concerns that he wasn't playing cooperatively with other children or talking as much as his peers. Instead, he was still focused on his own interests.

However, Jay was not interested in the 'expected' toys his peers were playing with. When Jay was around seven, his Dad bought him a game console. Again, Jay didn't play with his console in a conventional way. He became interested in how the games were made, leading him to discover coding. Looking back over Jay's play journey, he had always been interested in patterns of instructions, first with trains, then lifts and then traffic lights. His family often say that he has effectively been coding since he was born. Because Jay was encouraged to play his own way, he was able to find an interest where his creativity can now be seen clearly by others. He has also found friends who love coding and is making peer-to-peer social connections.

At no point was Jay made to feel concerned or strange about his own interests by his parents, and allowing this natural progression has allowed him to follow the things he loved. His autistic play and interests were respected and considered valid and important. Families of autistic children often discuss the lack of road map for their children, so following their own parental instinct is often much harder. There are still so many websites and professionals who advise on how children 'should' play. But the above scenario shows that all play is investigative and meaningful.

People unfamiliar with autistic styles of play, which are often not based on spoken communication, have historically drawn erroneous conclusions that autistic children play incorrectly. For example, a parallel play that continues beyond age-expected points in development can be framed as a 'red flag', but on closer inspection of parallel play, there can be a lot of observation, learning, modelling, and non-verbal communication happening.

Some years ago, in my early teaching days, I met a four-year-old girl called Nima at a nursery class. I remember the nursery explaining that they were looking to encourage Nima to display very typical types of socialising. At the time, I was not the main teacher and was given the opportunity to spend time with Nima, particularly to scaffold her skills. The nursery gave me the following instructions for supporting her.

We would like her to speak to her peers more, make eye contact more, and stop playing so much by herself because she is very isolated. Also, she hits out sometimes at other children, so we want that to stop.

I was told that she probably would not interact with me but that I should try to talk to her to encourage her reciprocal conversation skills. What follows is how this interaction played out. I called on my experience to support Nima in building a connection. I knew that having a safe key adult would be vital for Nima to be able to build further connections.

I watched little Nima engrossed in her game; she chatted to herself, happily moving items from the playground into a pile in a small wooden house. I sat close to her game but not so close as to impose, and I kept my gaze away from Nima. Nima had a little pile of items she had collected, and I began to show interest in her pile, not touching it, just looking over it. I did not make eye contact with Nima but smiled at her glorious pile of items. Nima noticed and looked at me as I continued to show interest in her things and what she was doing. She carried on, but she would come a little closer each time I smiled, not directly at Nima, but at her pile of precious items.

At one point, another child tried to take one of Nima's items from her pile. Her little face filled with anguish as she saw the boy reach for the item. I asked him if he could use a different item because these were very precious and important items that Nima was playing with. He nodded, put it back, and ran off. Nima's whole body noticeably relaxed. Then she came right up to me, picked up a small wooden box, and gave it to me. I smiled a broad smile (still not making eye contact) and walked over to her pile; I gestured to Nima's pile and said, 'On here?' She nodded. I put the item on the pile, and Nima clapped and laughed. She ran off to get more items to hand to me to put onto her pile.

The next day, when I arrived, Nima ran over and walked close by me. She watched as I said hello to the other children, and then I gave my full attention to her play. Again, she was playing her own game with water and blocks, which she was moving around. Nima would flick her eyes up to my face and then away again; we played together for a long time with the blocks. Nima was happy when one or two children would join her near the water, but any more than that, and she became noticeably tense. When a big group of children came over, she quickly left, pushing one child out of the way to escape. She looked worriedly at me and pulled my sleeve to bring me with her. We moved to the playhouse, and she again began grabbing items to make her pile; she was not smiling at first, and I wondered if she was still tense from all the children at the water table. I went with her and picked up an item; tentatively, I said, 'On here?' gesturing to her pile. Her smile returned, and we spent quite some time gathering items; Nima giggled as we played together.

Throughout my time with Nima, I did not force eye contact. Our eye contact was fleeting but also a sign that she relaxed into engaging with me. I did not force peer play as she needed a person (an adult) who could understand the rules of her play; the other children would need lots of scaffolding to play with Nima and respect her needs. I did not expect speech. We played a lovely game, building rapport without speech. I also did not reprimand her for pushing the other child but supported her need for space. For Nima to feel safe, it would be helpful for the other children to understand that they should not crowd her, which would need to be facilitated by an adult. I could see that Nima wanted to socialise, but she and her peers would need adult support to play in a way that Nima and another child could enjoy. Nima was in a nursery surrounded by children who were loud and unpredictable and were all socialising through speech. Expecting Nima to slot into such play was unfair to Nima and to the other children, as it could inevitably lead to difficulties due to the double empathy problem.

Forced spoken social exchanges based on 'expected' play can override autistic natural stages of development. Requiring a child to use eye contact during play can be off-putting for an autistic child, breaking them out of their creative process. The Early Years Foundation Stage (EYFS) handbook has a number of targets based on shared play. Autistic children might appear to fall at the first hurdle when they do not engage as expected. However, these targets are often wholly inappropriate and fail to value divergent types of play, socialising, and communication.

There is a difference between scaffolding learning and forced expectations. Scaffolding play means you meet the child where they are and support their skills while respecting their play style and seeking to develop skills as a co-facilitator. Scaffolding an autistic child looks different from supporting a non-autistic child. Removing expectations and joining their style of play is often beneficial.

Autistic play, whether lining items up, licking, touching, collecting, exploring, or investigating, is valid and important. Autistic children use play to build their understanding of the world through their own neurosensory profile. It is the systems and policies built around expected age-related targets that are flawed, not autistic children's style of play and communication.

PART SEVEN:
AUTISTIC TRAITS VERSUS EXPECTED TARGETS

This part will delve into the complex interplay between autistic traits and society's conventional expectations and targets, particularly in educational settings. To create an autistic-friendly society where all children can truly thrive, it is crucial to address and acknowledge the barriers many autistic children encounter. By identifying these obstacles, we can effectively work towards eliminating them.

Autistic children's developmental journeys often differ from traditional paths, leading to many unique talents and challenges. By making challenges explicit within the framework of age-related expectations, it becomes evident that typical societal expectations frequently do not align with the requirements of autistic children.

This part is organised to consider different traits often associated with autism. Each section offers a reframing of these traits through a neurosensory lens.

Access to non-literal language and meaning

Socially constructed knowledge is fed to children through a web of social interactions and cultural influences that shape their perceptions, beliefs, and understanding of reality. The messages children receive can also shape their ideas about themselves. Language serves as a fundamental building block in this process. It is the way knowledge is shared within communities. Language transfers values, biases and expectations. Children absorb language and its nuances from the earliest stages of development, internalising social norms and expectations. Shared language creates a collective understanding (groupthink) and instils social conditioning.

Simply put, spoken words, tone of voice, gestures and facial expressions marry to send messages to children. Take, for example, the words, 'I am so happy'. When accompanied by a genuine smile and corresponding gestures, these words mean a person is incredibly happy. The same words convey sarcasm when the 'so' is emphasised ('I am *so* happy') and combined with an exasperated facial expression. The words are the same, but the underlying meaning has changed. This nuance takes time for all young children to comprehend.

Comprehension of nuance is considered an age-related skill; non-literal language is thought to embed from approximately age five through to age nine. In truth, an understanding of non-literal language is not based on age but on speech comprehension. Children usually pick it up when they become fluent speakers. Prior to this stage, children learn the meanings of words, how they combine into phrases, and, eventually, sentences. They also acquire the ability to convey meaning through these sentences. This is the nuts-and-bolts stage of learning a language and is the same process one goes through when learning any other language. It is necessary to learn the nuts and bolts of the language before you can use that language in a nuanced way. To understand and use nuance, speech must be so fluent that it is second nature.

For autistic children, the nuts-and-bolts stage of learning a spoken language can be complex. They may not hear as many words or pick up as much contextual meaning as their peers. This is compounded by the presence of potential barriers to accessing facial cues, gestures, and tone of voice. For instance, some children with sensory abundance lip-read for assistance, and a child who relies on lip-reading might find it difficult to observe cues and gestures. Similarly, a child who isolates auditory input to focus on monoprocessing a person's voice might overlook visual cues. Additionally, discerning changes in tone of voice could be challenging in a noisy environment. These factors can all serve as obstacles to grasping nuanced layers of meaning.

Judgement, expectations and sarcasm are all conveyed through speech and body language. However, as previously discussed, autistic children may experience reduced or sporadic access to speech. Autistic children's nuts-and-bolts stage of learning language may look quite different from that of their peers. They might build meaning through exploring textures and embed learning about those textures. They might pick up on less verbal and more visual input building these into mini-films. Throughout this process, autistic children probably won't be as influenced by the ideas and expectations of the people around them.

Temple Grandin, the autistic scientist, did not speak until she was three and a half and clearly remembers being focused on visual patterns. As an adult, her brain scans showed that the visual circuitry in her brain extended beyond that seen in most people's brains. Temple has a strong long-term visual memory but has always had challenges remembering spoken information. Her pattern spotting, information gathering, and conceptual knowledge were built around her first language (accessing the things she could see over the things she could hear). Speech did not come naturally to Temple, and she was given speech lessons. Her speech journey was slow, and she stayed at the nuts-and-bolts stage for some time. During this period, she built conceptual knowledge by observing how things work.

At first, Temple's understanding of the world was quite literal, but her image-based memory expanded over time, allowing her to apply non-literal concepts to her thinking. She found that converting abstract ideas into pictorial analogies helped her grasp complex concepts more effectively. For instance, she visualised her immune system as a military base with soldiers, allowing her to understand its functioning better. This ability made her highly adept at using metaphors and similes to express herself. Despite her skills in understanding some figurative language, Temple still faced challenges with sarcasm. She attributes this difficulty to her thinking in pictures, as sarcasm does not easily translate to her visual language.

James is an autistic young person who mostly thinks in words; he is clear about how the translation process from speech to written words affects his access to non-literal language. Here, he reflects on a situation when he failed to recognise that his friend was employing sarcasm.

I am always very focused on the structure of sentences. I see the sentences in my mind as people say them, noticing the grammatical rules and then thinking about the different words they could have chosen, like a sort of synonym Filofax. I know that in conversations, a reply is expected. There is so much going on in my brain, and I often just respond with a genuine answer to the question being asked. It is only when all the people around me laugh that I realise the person is either being sarcastic or wasn't expecting the answer I gave.

(James, autistic young person)

However, it is not the case that all autistic people struggle with non-literal language. Many autistic people become well-versed in sarcasm, but this is usually after years of embedding. Rachel said she was a visual and tactile learner who learned through observing and recreating social patterns.

I was a real people watcher; people fascinated me. When I was younger, I was always trying to copy other people's clothes and actions. I remember very clearly when I first used sarcasm. I watched my older brother using a sarcastic tone of voice and thought it would be funny to try it. I was probably around nine or ten. I was given a book as a present and was not very happy with it. In front of my whole family, I said, 'Thanks, I really love it.' I used a sarcastic tone and made all my cousins laugh, but my parents were furious. They marched me away and reprimanded me, saying I should know better at my age than to be rude when I was given a present. I remember feeling so confused; I had only tried to copy my older brother - but had got the context completely wrong.

(Rachel, autistic adult)

Explicitly teaching autistic children non-literal language can be useful and fun. We did this with Jay using his first languages of writing and visuals. There is a great book called *It Is Raining Cats and Dogs*[80] that has funny visual representations of idioms. It is useful to consider

---

80   Barton, M. (2012). It's raining cats and dogs: an autism spectrum guide to the confusing world of idioms, metaphors, and everyday expressions. London ; Philadelphia: Jessica Kingsley Publishers.

how we scaffold autistic understanding of non-literal language and their grasp of social norms while not placing unrealistic expectations on them to intrinsically 'know' these nuanced elements within communication.

In the above examples, the nuts-and-bolts process of learning about speech-based nuance sets these people's experiences apart from the experiences of their similarly aged peers. This nuts-and-bolts stage also impacts access to social constructs. Socially constructed ideas include how children should behave, why they need to follow the rules, how they keep safe, etc. These are rules society deems necessary and are passed on to children through speech and gestures.

Take a scenario such as a child joining a nursery setting. There is often an array of rules to be communicated. When rules are mostly reinforced through speech, autistic children are at a disadvantage. If a child does not have consistent access to speech, it is not easy for them to access these rules. If they do access the words, they have to translate these through their first language to make sense of the rules and *then* understand that these rules change in different contexts: It is okay to shout in the playground but not in the classroom, for example. It is important to note that such rules are socially constructed and arbitrary. Autistic children who come to these rules later may well see some rules as nonsensical and question why they are in place. For example, an autistic child might be told they must learn to eat with a knife and fork, but they can eat a burger and chips with their fingers. They might be told never to lie but then be told they should pretend they like a present to spare another person's feelings.

For autistic children, embedding societal rules and expectations can take longer and can be confusing. It also means that autistic children are, in some ways, less constrained by societal expectations. This can present as autistic children not following behavioural expectations or social norms, which can attract judgement from others in society. Often, autistic children might appear to behave like younger children when they are, in fact, behaving appropriately for their own stage of development and communication.

If and when autistic children pass the nuts-and-bolts stage, it can feel like they are learning on the job. This is because young children often receive explicit teaching around concepts in their early years. They will be taught about crossing the road, not talking to strangers, being kind, etc. Autistic children who are trying to follow social rules without this explicit support can be seen as getting things 'wrong'.

Social norms are so rigid, and I think this is a feature of humans; non-neurodiverse humans fit into very tight social norms, and I think if you are a bit out of that, people don't like it.

(Jules, autistic adult)

The above examples underscore the importance of recognising and appreciating diverse communication journeys in the context of autistic first and second languages. It is often expected that autistic children should change their way of thinking and communicating to 'fit in' with society. However, teaching society to accept autistic ways of being would allow autistic children to express themselves genuinely.

Age-related Social and Emotional Expectations

'I am an autistic adult. I cannot read a clock, I do not know multiplication, and I have trouble tying my shoes. I am a law graduate and hold a corporate job. The ability to tie your shoelaces does not determine your success.'

Mikaela Ackerman, *Edge of the Playground*[81]

The EYFS[82] document, which covers personal, social and emotional development (PSED), contains a perplexing contradiction regarding the approach to child development. While acknowledging that children progress and learn at their own pace, the framework also

---

81   Ackerman, M. and Lynn, M. (2019). The Edge of The Playground: Two Stories One Journey: A Mother and Daughter's Memoir of Autism From Childhood to Adulthood.

82   Department for Education (2021). Early years foundation stage statutory framework (EYFS). [online] GOV.UK. Available at: https://www.gov.uk/government/publications/early-years-foundation-stage-framework--2.

suggests that concerns should be raised if a child 'falls behind' in prime areas. Under PSED, goals such as self-regulation, managing self and building relationships are listed. The belief that children should display specific social and emotional traits at certain ages is flawed. Children's social and emotional development closely tracks their access to a useful communication tool.

This can create challenges for young autistic children, who may follow a different social and emotional trajectory compared to their non-autistic peers. This emphasis on assessment and reaching predefined Early Learning Goals can lead to autistic children being perceived as not progressing as expected. I cannot stress this enough: children cannot 'progress' the way a statutory document expects them to. They are little humans who can only progress in the way that their little human bodies and brains enable them to.

With regards to building relationships, children typically gain access to the inner thoughts and feelings of other children when they can listen to and comprehend those feelings. Until this stage is reached, they are often characterised as being at an egocentric developmental stage, primarily focused on their own wants and needs. It is important to note that autistic children, even if they do not have access to speech, can advance beyond this stage through visual observation and by employing alternative communication systems (see socially constructed empathy).

Other Early Learning Goals are based on the behaviours

expected around a certain age. When an autistic child takes longer to understand personal space and boundaries, engages in toy-snatching, or hits out at another child, it is their age that prevents them from receiving equity. Where a younger child would be supported in developing these skills, autistic children can be flagged as acting inappropriately. That is not to say they should be considered similar to younger children. Autistic children are full of conceptual learning; it's just that their conceptual learning may not follow the expected patterns.

Autistic children may also display behaviours that challenge because they are at a developmental stage where these behaviours serve them. For example, some young children enjoy throwing things or kicking things over and autistic children may do this for longer than their similarly aged peers. Or they may enjoy certain sensory feedback from unexpected behaviours such as breaking things or headbanging. In some cases, head banging may be the result of too much brain activity, where the child is trying to dampen that activity. It may also be a form of communication or a sensory and developmental need. These stages of development can be very unnerving for parents and teachers of autistic children; the best thing may be to allow these behaviours in places where the child cannot hurt themselves or others, for example, throwing things in a space with no other children around. It is essential to work out whether such behaviours are fulfilling a sensory need or whether there is a different underlying need. Obviously, if these behaviours signify anxiety or trauma, then different supports would be needed to reduce said trauma.

Children are expected to embed concepts around avoiding danger. Most of us would not cross a road by walking out into oncoming traffic; we understand that to be safe, we should wait at the roadside or cross at a crossing. This might seem like an intrinsic skill, but waiting at the roadside is a learned behaviour children acquire through observation and spoken re-enforcement. Some children lack conceptual awareness of dangers, and this creates a number of problems for the families who experience it. Autistic children can elope (they wander away from their caregiver, home or school), or they might remove their seatbelt when a car is moving. Parents are often expected to manage this themselves, and there are very few affordable safety options for older children.

Children who are not as tuned into verbal concepts require more time to reach milestones, particularly in the context of social and behavioural expectations. To create a more inclusive and supportive environment, it is crucial to develop policies that reflect this understanding, where their traits are acknowledged as appropriate for their stage of development, and suitable accommodations and support are provided to facilitate their progress.

Autistic divergent social and emotional development can manifest in various ways, such as:

- Developing some skills later than their similarly aged

peers

- A lack of awareness of danger
- Attaining self-care targets later than peers
- Watching cartoons or playing with toys typically intended for younger children
- Feeling anxious when exposed to uncomfortable parts of films
- Feeling anxious when reading books with challenging themes like death or peril
- Asking numerous questions about concepts that non-autistic children have already grasped
- Appearing emotionally sensitive or insensitive
- Appearing to misread social cues and rules
- Preferring to interact with a social group that shares similar traits
- Playing alone to avoid the challenges of social communication with non-autistic peers

To best support autistic children, settings should assess their readiness and introduce concepts when children are socially and emotionally prepared. This removes the current system of viewing their progress as delayed. Children may also need to be taught some concepts in multi-sensory ways, taking their sensory profile and first language into account.

Socially constructed expected empathy

Although the initial stages of empathy are based on mirroring behaviours, the latter stages are, in many ways, a taught concept. Children are not born with an innate deep empathy for others; they develop empathy over time. Empathy is split into different stages, which children move between. Initially, children react to the pain of others as if they themselves were feeling that pain and then offer the comfort they themselves would like. This is considered an egocentric stage where the child only understands the self. Then, around the age of three, children begin to understand that other children have feelings different from their own and can offer comfort in a non-egocentric way. The final stage is when children understand that outside factors such as biases and hierarchy can impact children's well-being.

The initial stage of empathy, where a child mirrors another child's responses, is primarily based on observation. The child literally mirrors the crying child's response. As empathy develops, speech becomes a key component of learning how another child feels. These learnings are fed through reciprocal conversations alongside observation.

An autistic child who is engaged in picking up visual patterns may experience the mirroring of empathetic responses much more keenly. When a child is hurt, they would also cry or complain of being hurt. This can be mistaken as the autistic child seeking attention when it is actually a mirrored empathetic approach. This can become an autistic go-to way of showing empathy. Many autistic adults discuss the fact that they show empathy by sharing or mirroring similar stories. But this is often not well understood by non-autistic people; apparently (and I had to look this up), non-autistic empathy involves:

- focusing on the other person, not yourself
- ensuring the person feels heard by repeating back their important points
- learning more about their situation by asking questions

For autistic children, the above would take quite a bit of mental load. It is not in alignment with their monotropic traits and would lead to a rather stilted interaction, where the autistic child would be following an 'expected empathy' script. A significant factor contributing to the misconception that autistic individuals lack empathy is the fundamental difference in how autistic and non-autistic people communicate and perceive empathy.

Autistic children may offer a hurt or crying child comfort in the way they themselves would like to be comforted. Again, this can diverge from the expected – where a non-autistic child might offer a hug or touch, an autistic child might offer the injured party a toy or try to stop the crying through other means. It becomes important to consider the reason behind autistic actions instead of interpreting these actions through a non-autistic lens. An autistic child might also show signs that they are inquisitive about what is happening, moving very close to a child without seemingly showing any empathy. However, this should not be interpreted as a lack of care but instead a lack of conceptual understanding of what is happening, where the autistic child is using exploratory tactics to understand the situation better.

Autistic children experiencing sensory abundance may be too overwhelmed to show expected empathy. For example, in a nursery setting, sensory abundance is so overwhelming for them that another child crying just adds to that input. Their instinct is not to mirror that child; instead, their instinct is to get away from the increased painful input. This can, understandably, override an autistic child's capacity to show expected empathy for other children, and could be misinterpreted as a problem with self-regulating. Paradoxically, an autistic child who thinks mainly in words may find it hard to connect to their emotional responses and the emotional responses of others in an expected way. Instead, they display something called cognitive empathy, where they understand that the other child needs support, but they do not *feel* their feelings.

Non-autistic children can lack empathy for autistic children's experiences because they cannot put themselves in an autistic child's shoes. For example, it is hard to imagine why an autistic child becomes so upset about sensory overwhelm or about losing control. Often, an autistic child's emotional response to seemingly small things can be hard for others to understand. In this way, autistic sensory anxiety and a lack of understanding can serve as barriers to social connection.

As children progress into the final stage of empathy, characterised by their desire to help and support other children, they gain cognitive autonomy to decide whether they will offer assistance or support to another child. The flip side of this level of cognition is that children enter the stage of 'groupthink', which can drive children to exclude, bully and judge others. This suggests that autistic children can become highly vulnerable when their peers of similar age develop this understanding. At this point, some children may opt for inclusion and acceptance of autistic peers, while others might unfairly judge autistic traits and consequently exclude them. As autistic children may still be at the nuts-and-bolts stage of language and at the earlier stages of empathy, this type of rejection can be distressing and confusing. In many cases, autistic children will seek out safe friendships with children who understand them.

Socially constructed emotions

Emotions are not fixed or uniform; they are experienced and interpreted differently by each individual. This holds true for both autistic and non-autistic individuals. Autistic children may construct their emotional responses in ways unique to their sensory experiences and conceptual understanding. What brings joy and happiness to an autistic child might differ from what evokes similar emotions in a non-autistic child. For example, an autistic child may find immense pleasure in exploring an object, triggering the release of dopamine and leading to attachment to such items. Alternatively, they may find comfort and joy in being in a tight space, as the pressure on their body brings relief to their muscles, whether they are feeling tight or loose.

On the other hand, inputs that trigger a trauma response in an autistic child may be puzzling to people who don't grasp the concept of autistic Neurosensory Divergence. For instance, when an autistic child associates loud noises with pain, their reaction to potential loud sounds is grounded in the belief that they are in immediate danger of harm. To visualise this, imagine emotions as a dial, with one end representing intense fear and the other end representing intense joy. Autistic children who experience sensory abundance are more prone to experience emotions towards either end of the dial, meaning they do not go through life with the same emotional range as most of their peers. This reframes autistic emotional responses as appropriate responses to their experiences due to them taking in more sensory information.

The impact of these emotional experiences on autistic children is often poorly understood. They are frequently expected to display emotions in the same manner as non-autistic children. Autistic big emotions can be framed as inappropriate and odd. For instance, a child who continuously cries at nursery might be labelled overly sensitive. Instead of recognising that their emotional response could be a genuine reaction to sensory pain, it is instead framed as a lack of regulation skills in autistic children. Autistic children are taught to match the size of their emotional reaction to the problem. However, this assumes that the person supporting the autistic child understands the size of the problem for the child.

They may be taught to subdue their emotion if it is not considered an appropriate response. It can be perplexing for autistic children to be encouraged to suppress their feelings, as their natural responses are disregarded and diminished. Consequently, this can impact their internal emotional awareness and self-understanding. If a child is taught not to embrace their feelings, it can hinder their ability to articulate and describe their emotional state accurately.

Several scenarios can make it challenging for autistic individuals to explain and comprehend their emotions. Prolonged trauma, particularly intense trauma, can lead to emotional blunting, resulting in an inability to experience the full range of emotions. Additionally, because sensory trauma is poorly understood, autistic children may repeatedly encounter distressing situations in their early years before they can communicate their distress effectively.

Moreover, their emotional responses to these situations can be complex. For instance, an autistic child may adore school but despise the bullying they face on the playground, or they may enjoy going to a concert with friends but feel overwhelmed by the loudness and commotion. This complexity can lead to experiencing multiple emotions simultaneously. If speech is not an autistic child's first language, expressing this complexity could be challenging.

Teaching emotions to autistic children

Autistic children can experience challenges when describing their own emotions. This could be because the narrative around them at school might be the emotional experiences of a non-autistic child. I will use an example of a recent piece of homework that came home with Jay to illustrate this point. In the homework, the children were asked to choose the face that best matched a given description. One of the faces depicted a child labelled *bored*, and the corresponding description included:

- Looking away from the teacher
- Looking down at the floor or up at the ceiling
- Fiddling with things

This description of a bored child could also fit the behaviour of an engaged autistic child. Autistic children often need to look away from visual input and engage in fidgeting to process and access spoken information effectively. This can lead to confusion for autistic children because they are being taught that their autistic emotional state is equivalent to a different emotional state in a non-autistic person.

When autistic children are taught about emotions, they are often given a very surface understanding of emotions. This is helpful in the early stages of teaching and learning, where they might be given a picture of a smiling face and be taught that it means *happy*. It can become problematic when teaching stops at the basics. When autistic children are not taught about the nuances of emotional states and body language, they are left with a very surface understanding of their own emotions and the emotions of others, on the level of, 'When a child smiles, they are happy'. Some autistic children may embed this concept in a scripted literal way and take this as a fact, but it is not always true. Children grimace when hurt; they sometimes smile when being unkind; sometimes, they smile to cover up the fact that they are sad. This can leave autistic children vulnerable when socialising as they may misread cues or miss that children are being unkind to them.

Autistic children would benefit from revisiting these concepts regularly, while also validating their own autistic emotional responses. If we do not offer ongoing affirming scaffolding of emotions, it is unfair to expect autistic children to learn by osmosis.

Social constructs and gender

Rules surrounding gender have been passed down through generations, shaping societal perceptions of what is considered appropriate or inappropriate for each gender. These norms can be fed through various channels, including conversations, books and media representations. As discussed earlier, autistic children may not be as engaged in these representations, as they often focus more on their own interests rather than adhering to spoken cues. Consequently, some autistic children may not engage in play that aligns with expected binary gendered norms and may not identify with these expected ways of being.

Autistic children may also come to grasp the explicit concept of gender identity later than their non-autistic peers, and they may raise questions about their own identity. When a four- or five-year-old enquires about their identity, they are frequently provided with a binary response that they are either a boy or a girl. Often, play grows around these binary ideas of gender. However, socially constructed ideas of what a girl or boy 'should' do or be may not necessarily align with the autistic child's authentic experience.

I did not want to play families like the other girls. I wanted to play with dinosaurs. I had every dinosaur under the sun. I loved to roar and run around. I did not like playing families at all. But I did want friends, so I would play families because the other girls did not want to play dinosaurs.

(Eleanor, autistic child)

There is growing evidence that gender variance is more prevalent in autistic communities. Experiences and interactions shape identities. Having divergent access to early speech-based communication means that, for many autistic children, gender norms and expectations are likely to be less embedded during early childhood. That is not to say that autistic children are not constructing ideas around their own identity. They very much will be. Autistic children and adults are often positioned as not 'seeing the bigger picture' because of their focused interests, but many autistic people often see *more* of the bigger picture. For example, when it comes to gender, many do not feel as hemmed in by the binary idea of gender conformity. Autistic people are much more likely to question socially constructed concepts, including ideas around gender.

Wenn Lawson, a transgender autistic man, discusses this topic in the book *The Awesome Autistic Go-To Guide*[83], pointing out that many autistic people struggle

---

83   Purkis, Y. and Masterman, T. (2020). The Awesome Autistic Go-To Guide. Jessica Kingsley Publishers.

to connect with the predetermined societal expectations of who they 'should' be based on gender norms and some feel confused as they attempt to conform to the gender assigned to them at birth. Like every aspect of being autistic, understanding one's own gender and sexuality can be a complex journey. When autistic children do not conform to societal norms, it can lead to judgement and derision. This pressure to conform can result in masking, where a child hides their actual wants and needs to avoid rejection.

The social construction of autistic rigid thinking

Autistic children are often framed as rigid thinkers. The truth is *all* humans are pattern-based, rigid thinkers. Most of us display these behaviours because they are practical and give us a sense of well-being and control. These patterns are often hard to spot because most humans in society follow similar behavioural patterns. For example, we mostly eat similar things for breakfast, many of us eat meals around the same times each day, and many of us have a set pattern of working. These behavioural patterns (or routines) make us feel like we know what is coming next, and this sense of sameness can be reassuring. We also have some patterns of behaviour that reduce our cognitive load; for example, most daily jobs include similar tasks within a specific industry. It would feel pretty unnerving if you were a teacher one day, then the next day, without warning, you were expected to be an accountant.

Another example of a pattern many people in the UK tend to follow is related to national holidays. Many people have become accustomed to celebrating Easter and Christmas at set times of the year whether they are religious or not; if either were suddenly cancelled, this might cause emotions connected to that change. In autistic children, the need for sameness appears more pronounced because it is built around their sensory profile. For instance, an autistic child might strongly identify with always having a blue cup in a similar way that others might connect with the significance of always having holidays like Christmas or Easter at the same time each year.

To avoid potential pain and trauma, autistic children may be understandably more inclined towards sameness. However, sameness is hard to sustain, and many autistic children will struggle with this part of their life. They often look to their parents or caregivers to manage this, and many parents become adept at sticking to routines. Children with less access to spoken language can find this part of their profile particularly challenging.

Controlling situations

Autistic children might seek to 'control' situations for a number of reasons. They might employ tactics of avoidance or control to evade possible traumas. Autistic children may be at an egocentric stage of language and social development, where they are focused on their own wants and needs, and so might control play to meet their own needs. When asked to stop an activity, they may be in a monotropic focus tunnel, and leaving a joyful moment feels like an intrusion into their happiness. In situations where they feel at a disadvantage (such as playing a game or sport), autistic children might change the rules of a game to ensure they have equity within that game.

In Pathological Demand Avoidance (an autistic profile characterised by avoiding everyday demands), this drive for autonomy can be all-encompassing. PDA children can appear resistant to many activities, often themselves not fully grasping why they are avoidant. It may be the case that attempting to live a life steeped in 'expected' goals is actually at odds with their autistic profile. Even activities that may be enjoyable in part will probably include challenges around sensory and social demands. Again, understanding that NSD profiles might mean autistic children need to access life on their own terms can be very useful. It is important to try to understand the reasons autistic children try to engineer situations to meet their needs, in order to support them through transitions and to offer equitable adjustments.

Physical development

Some autistic children have divergent motor abilities, and this can alter developmental timelines. Tasks that many children begin to coordinate in their early years, such as navigating around a classroom, self-dressing, tying shoelaces and so on, might not be possible or might be possible later in some autistic children's developmental journey. School targets around handwriting and sports need to be looked at to ensure equitable targets are in place. Although some schools do use inclusive practices, this is not currently commonplace. Pressure can be placed on autistic children and their families to develop skills alongside their peers, and this can cause ongoing trauma for autistic children.

According to the Equality Act[84], a disability is a physical or mental impairment that substantially and adversely affects normal daily activities. Therefore, autistic children who face challenges in developing fine and gross motor skills could be considered disabled under the Act and should be offered reasonable (or rather necessary) adjustments. Unfortunately, motor differences are not always recognised as a disability in autistic children.

Therapies available to support autistic motor skills encompass physiotherapy and occupational therapy.

---

84   GOV.UK (2010). Definition of Disability under the Equality Act 2010. [online] GOV.UK. Available at: https://www.gov.uk/defini tion-of-disability-under-equality-act-2010.

Autistic children can derive significant benefits from affirming physiotherapy and occupational therapy, which can aid in the development of physical co-regulation strategies and can scaffold motor skills. Nonetheless, it is crucial that these therapies are administered in a way that caters to the child's individual needs and abilities, rather than trying to push them into standardised goals.

In early years settings and schools, it would be advantageous to establish individualised fine and gross motor skill targets for autistic children. Implementing such targets can pose challenges in settings built around age-related expectations, particularly in classrooms with whole-class teaching. Nevertheless, I have witnessed instances where schools have effectively embraced inclusion and equity by pioneering innovative solutions.

Furthermore, there are numerous sports clubs organised by charities and local councils that offer inclusive sessions. These opportunities can prove invaluable, fostering both physical and social growth in the lives of autistic children. One such social enterprise is Action Attainment,[85] which not only puts on sessions but also educates on how their inclusive sessions can be incorporated into schools. Families of autistic children are crying out for more inclusive out-of-school physical activities for their children.

85   Action Attainment. (n.d.). Action Attainment. [online] Available at: https://www.action-attainment.com/ [Accessed 23 Aug. 2023].

Busy brains

To consider only behavioural responses in autistic profiles is to negate the underlying processes of those profiles. Although the neurodiversity movement has moved the autism narrative forward to consider how divergent brains create behaviours, the autistic divergent body-brain connection is rarely discussed. Neurosensory Divergence asks that we consider how sensory stimuli impact autistic children's bodies.

Over time, autistic children may experience more sensory pain and social trauma than most children. These experiences often trigger the fight or flight response, a well-known physiological reaction. For autistic children, this stress response can become a frequent occurrence, affecting their overall well-being. The parasympathetic nervous system plays a role in dampening this stress response, but chronic stress is challenging to alleviate. A crucial aspect of this process is the check-in stage, where the body assesses if the stressor is still present. This means the body and brain scan to see if the potential danger remains. If the threat persists, stress levels remain heightened.

Autistic children in busy or demanding environments may find themselves stuck in a cycle where their stress levels continue to rise due to sensory stimulation. This prolonged exposure to overwhelming situations can exacerbate their stress response, leading to significant challenges in managing sensory input effectively. Neurosensory Divergence means that autistic children may experience this state continuously throughout the day. This progression happens so rapidly that, at times, they may not even be aware of this ongoing process.

James, an autistic thirteen-year-old, experiences sensory overload:

> *At school, I just seemed to lose it really quickly. Feelings kind of rushed over me sometimes in class. I think maybe I felt stressed most of the time at school, but I didn't really register it because it was a feeling that was always there, bubbling under the surface.*

Another stressor that can affect autistic children is being in an environment primarily reliant on speech-based input. Autistic children who struggle to access and comprehend spoken information may be constantly on high alert. This perpetual state of heightened alertness can trigger autistic perfectionism, where they attempt to conceal their struggles and challenges.

Heidi, an autistic adult, eloquently conveys how she felt during such moments:

> *[I was] trying not to humiliate myself, I think, because I was especially scared of the teachers who would do calling upon kids for answers and stuff. So, I was extra vigilant during those lessons. And would really, really hate having those teachers; I just had no trust in them at all.*

Providing autistic children with the opportunity to

comprehend why they experience these challenges and equipping them with the tools and opportunities to balance their internal systems could prove invaluable. Autistic children are not inherently bad self-regulators; they simply have more challenges to cope with than most children. Empowering them with support and understanding can make a significant positive difference in their lives.

We all stim

Understanding the intensity of autistic sensory experiences and gaining insight into their inner workings can shed light on the difficulties autistic children encounter in maintaining a harmonious brain-body connection. There is much more internal activity to balance! It is well known that physical movement triggers hormonal changes and can balance the electrical and chemical processes associated with stress responses. Studies have shown that contracting muscles can help to release chemicals such as myokines molecules (dubbed hope molecules) into the bloodstream, crossing the blood-brain barrier and creating an antidepressant/anti-anxiety effect. The best way to keep this cycle going is through repetitive movements. This includes fine motor muscles in the ear, the eyes, and the fingers, as well as larger muscles in the legs and arms. Cyclical, repetitive activities help human bodies internally regulate elevated blood pressure, heart rate, breathing, and whole-body emotional responses (associated with that elevation).

These movements are known as self-stimulatory movements (stims). Autistic children may need more of these muscle contractions to regulate their internal state effectively, dampening the stress they experience throughout the day. Stimming is framed as an autistic trait, where a person uses repetitive movements to regulate or express feelings. It is undoubtedly true that autistic children will need more movement because (as I have discussed) they are experiencing more intense sensory input and cognitive load. But I do not see stimming as a requirement for only autistic bodies. Here, I want to introduce the concept that everybody stims. I do not mean in the sense that we all tap our feet or that we all bite our nails. I mean, as in the whole-body experience of stimming.

Playgrounds are built around many of the movements we consider 'autistic' stims. As a society, we know that children need and enjoy spinning, swinging, and jumping. It is a human trait to use rhythmical motion and movements to regulate. These activities involve repetitive movements, calming the body and creating a sense of well-being. But when children enter institutions, their natural inclination towards this behaviour is often controlled through constructed ideas of appropriate and inappropriate behaviour. Set times are allocated to movement as children move through nursery and then school. Children can run, skip, jump, dig, and so on during these times and all of these include repetitive movements. The time allocated for movement decreases as children get older.

Most children fall in line, containing their movement when directed to; whether this is through a natural maturation process or conditioning is up for debate. Autistic children have a double whammy in these situations: they need more movement to regulate, *and* many are not consistently accessing spoken behavioural expectations. This requirement to contain their stim behaviours is further compounded by other children who can tease and bully children who act in unexpected ways.

Chloé Hayden, an autistic, ADHD disability rights activist, discusses this in her book *Different, Not Less*.[86] She says that as a young person, she was told to stop stimming and was taught to conform. She talks of forcing away her need to stim to avoid further bullying. It did not have the desired effect; attempting to override what her body naturally needed resulted in stored-up anxiety and behaviours that she could not control. Like many autistic children and young people who attempt to mask their natural traits, Chloé resorted to less healthy ways of suppressing her anxiety, such as scratching her skin and biting her lip. As discussed, removing autistic autonomy over their basic needs can create feelings of hopelessness at the loss of control.

I have often seen professionals discuss re-directing stims to more appropriate options for the classroom, but autistic children tell me that even this neglects to

---

86   Hayden, C. (2022). Different, Not Less. Allen & Unwin.

consider the purposeful nature of specific stims. For example, Josie, an autistic girl I mentored, told me that spinning helps her block out external sensory input while simultaneously calming her system, while a jumping stim helps her reconnect with her body.

If stim behaviours are a natural part of the lives of all young children, how do such behaviours cease to be a part of non-autistic adults' lives? The truth is that stim behaviours (repetitive movements) are a natural part of most everyday lives, well into adulthood, but are hidden in plain sight. As children age, this need for repetitive movements is often channelled through sports and hobbies. Everything from football to sewing uses repetitive movements. All these activities fulfil different needs, which continue into adulthood. A stressed person may participate in strenuous activities such as running, cycling, or playing squash, which all use repetitive movements. When a more relaxing repetitive stim is needed, a person might listen to music (with a repeated verse and chorus), or other relaxing stims might be knitting, painting, gardening – even sitting on a beach watching the waves gently flow in and out. We choose our stim based on the needs we are seeking to meet.

Autistic children (like all children) use stimming to help them balance internal processes and reduce anxiety created through hormonal imbalances. This is a human need. Autistic children may use more intense stim behaviours and need them more regularly, but they are simply fulfilling a human need. Seeing stimming as a natural part of human behaviour could remove stigma and create a greater understanding of the autistic need for movement.

PART EIGHT:
SETTINGS

NSD autistic children who are learning alongside their non-autistic peers can face challenges due to the way learning is traditionally organised and delivered. Alongside working within a standardised education, they are also navigating the social and sensory elements of settings. Many autistic children enjoy nursery and school, or they hold a strong desire to do so, but there can be barriers to that enjoyment. There are definitely ways we can accommodate more autistic children to thrive in our education system. Many schools and nurseries attain this goal by implementing innovative and unconventional approaches, showing that it is possible to offer an inclusive education within supportive environments for autistic children. The fact that these schools must step outside of current systems and policies in order to make targets and settings more equitable, seems to suggest that current systems and environments may not be optimal for all autistic children.

Early Years

Most Early Years settings in England are organised around a child-centred ethos of self-directed learning. Allowing children access to different learning resources throughout the day means they can find the things that most interest them. Teachers and support staff interact with children as facilitators of the child's learning. One way of assisting children in this process is called scaffolding. Scaffolding is a dynamic and effective method through which teachers provide targeted support to children as they explore and acquire new concepts or skills. In the instructional scaffolding model, teachers play a vital role in introducing fresh information and demonstrating problem-solving techniques to the children. This style of self-directed learning can encourage natural peer interaction and collaborative learning without the reliance on fluent speech.

Self-directed learning can foster critical thinking and nurture a deeper understanding of the subject matter. Activities can be thoughtfully tailored to cater to different learning styles, and what's intriguing is that children often make connections that span traditional subjects. Take, for instance, a child who builds a tower out of cardboard, striving to make it as tall as possible while carefully reinforcing its structure. In this seemingly simple activity, the child is not only experiencing the joy of creation but is also delving into scientific concepts and exploring the principles of balance and stability, understanding the effects of gravity on the tower's height, and learning about the properties of the materials they are using. This integrated approach to learning allows children to naturally connect various disciplines, fostering a holistic understanding of the world around them.

Early years settings now have more formal teaching than ever before, with separate sessions for maths and English. There is also tracking of children's subject knowledge. This style of learning caters more to the adults who wish to measure and compare students against standardised targets. Our education systems and structures also rely heavily on testing children's knowledge through written or spoken feedback. However, the type of deep learning that occurs in self-directed learning cannot be easily evaluated through standardised tests, especially when a child struggles to articulate their learning in spoken words. This does not mean that self-directed learning is suboptimal for the child: it is only suboptimal in a system that seeks to compare children.

Interest-driven learning can be a highly beneficial approach for many autistic children, as their alternative languages and unique and non-standardised ways of thinking enable them to make innovative discoveries. However, when these children are placed in nurseries and reception classes that follow rigid age-related expectations, they may face challenges on two fronts. Firstly, being judged based on these age-related targets can lead to undue pressure. Secondly, the sensory aspect of such settings can act as a significant barrier to their learning experience.

Nursery settings and playgroups often involve lots of sensory stimulation. Children are constantly moving around and making noise. While this environment might be enjoyable for non-autistic children, it can be overwhelming and unpredictable for an autistic child with minimal access to speech. To create a more inclusive and supportive learning environment, it is essential to acknowledge and accommodate the sensory needs of autistic children. Reducing sensory overload in these settings can make a significant difference in autistic children's ability to learn and thrive. This might involve providing quiet spaces where autistic children can let off steam alongside low arousal spaces where access to speech is optimised.

Dedicated staff who are inquisitive about autistic children and their learning journeys can build strong, cohesive connections. Early years practitioners are often adept at using non-speech-based resources, which can be really positive in aiding autistic learning access. Although early years settings offer the kind of education where autistic children can thrive, addressing sensory and social barriers is essential to meet the needs of autistic children.

Mainstream state schools

Once children transition to primary school in England, the emphasis on self-directed learning often decreases and teacher-led instruction becomes the primary mode of education. The shift from child-driven exploration to a more structured learning environment can present advantages and challenges. Teachers deliver lessons based on the targets outlined in the National Curriculum. This document serves as a guiding framework for primary and secondary schools; it sets out the subjects to be taught and the expected standards to be achieved by students.

Neurosensory learning profiles in mainstream schools

The National Curriculum was introduced in 1989 in England and Wales and aimed to promote uniformity and ensure a certain standard of education across the country. While it has brought some benefits, it is not without flaws. The targets set out in the National Curriculum are not structured around divergent pattern recognition or spiky learning profiles. This means that autistic children attending mainstream schools must work towards targets aimed at non-autistic children. During the 1980s and 1990s, parents were given a choice to educate their children in mainstream schools and the number of special schools declined significantly. Many autistic children were welcomed into these mainstream schools with the promise of high-quality teaching through inclusive practices. The clash between the standardisation of the National Curriculum and the diverse learning profiles of autistic children has since become apparent.

Unmet needs in a standardised education setting may not always be a 'special need' but a call for a more diverse and inclusive approach to learning. As long as education sticks to the current formula of a narrow type of education, there will continue to be children who are identified as not reaching standardised targets. Unconventional teaching should be an integral part of teaching and learning because, in every classroom, there will be many neurodivergent and neurosensory divergent children. I believe the answer is to elevate the opportunities for children to play to their strengths within their own sensory profile.

To explain my point, let me tell a story about myopia (near-sightedness).

Around 723 years ago, the first pair of glasses were invented, and 322 years ago, glasses started to be used by more people. How did people with myopia cope before this momentous invention? It is thought that people with myopia were placed in roles that suited their near-sightedness. Painting Bibles and illustrating manuscripts required great precision in creating tiny, detailed brushstrokes. The myopic person was not considered to have a disability. Instead, these were sought-out people who were viewed as skilled in their art.[87] In the modern day, myopia is seen as a trait that needs to be corrected by glasses. What has changed?

87   Gannon, M. (2019). How Did Nearsighted People Manage Before Glasses Were Invented? [online] livescience.com. Available at: https://www.livescience.com/65229-nearsighted-people-be fore-glasses-invented.html.

Around the same time as glasses became more sought-after, society became more literate. These two events were not a coincidence. There was a mismatch between the abilities of near-sighted people and the eyesight required for efficient reading. At this point, myopia was transformed into a disability (something that makes it more difficult for a person to complete certain activities). In this way, something considered a gift in one era becomes a disability in another era.

This idea that society constructs and deconstructs what constitutes celebrated abilities and disabilities is at the heart of why divergent learning profiles are often not valued as highly as expected or standardised learning profiles. Over time, vocational skills have been marginalised and are often dismissed as 'soft skills', while the focus has shifted towards prioritising 'core subjects' such as Mathematics, English, and Science. This shift means academic excellence is now associated with embedding specific patterns and codes. For neurosensory divergent children with spiky learning profiles, this is a big problem. Children destined to be artists, bakers, nurses, and coders (I could go on) might be drawn to pursuits outside this narrow view of a 'good education'. Tactile learners, visual learners, and even grapheme-based learners[88]*, through no fault of their own, might go through their entire school journey without having their talents fully recognised or rewarded. Even when autistic children do show abilities in the core

88   * Grapheme based learners – children who learn predominant-ly through the written word

subjects, their sensory divergence, access issues and communication differences might mean they cannot effectively show what they are capable of in mainstream classrooms.

In education, there can be talk of 'driving up standards' from the people in charge, especially when exam results in core areas fall below expectations. This often translates to an updated expectation that *all* children should demonstrate more knowledge of the core subjects at younger and younger ages or that exams should be made more challenging. For autistic children who are not necessarily accessing speech or following the same developmental trajectory as their similarly aged peers, this moving of the goalposts can be problematic. It can lead to more and more children falling below the 'expected' standard, only to be labelled as having learning difficulties. The socially constructed belief that all children should acquire knowledge at a similar age fails to celebrate the diversity of learning styles and the natural learning divergence that exists among children.

There is currently a crisis in the number of children requiring an Education Health Care Plan (EHCP). There are limited funds and there is a considerable backlog of children who are identified as needing support. It is probable that this crisis is indicative of the narrowing of academic expectations and the undervaluation of diverse learning styles. Neurosensory divergent children thrive when they can engage through their strengths and interests. A plethora of research states that a child-centred education, where children learn through intrinsic motivation, is the optimal way for many children to learn. Frequently, concerns are raised that self-directed learning might not be effective, as there is apprehension that children may overlook core skills. Yet these skills are introduced effectively through this method in the early years. I am not saying that core subjects are not important. Of course, they are, but they are not the *only* important subjects, and they will not feature as the most important learned skills in lots of children's lives.

Constant testing of these core subjects means that children are continually compared against one another. Comparing children and linking their worth to their ability to conform to a standardised education is less than optimal for neurosensory divergent children. Because of standardised testing, a child's ability to learn and retain information about highly valued subjects is considered the pinnacle of all school achievements.

Neurosensory divergent children often possess remarkable abilities to learn and retain extensive information. However, the value and recognition of their memory skills can be influenced by the specific nature of their neurosensory profile. When their memory is predominantly focused on tactile or image-driven activities, such as design technology or art, it may not be as highly appreciated or rewarded in traditional educational settings. If their memory centres around specific interests, such as memorising every Pokémon character or the names of animal species within a particular family, it is sometimes framed as a 'restricted interest' rather than a valuable memory skill. This double standard stems from socially constructed ideas about what society considers useful and important skills. For autistic children who learn and retain information divergently from the majority, a standardised curriculum built around non-autistic expected targets is often not optimal.

Memory and executive functioning

Autistic children have been described as lacking executive functioning, but as discussed, autistic memory can build around their pattern recognition and first languages. Many autistic children struggle to follow instructions, but how are these delivered? If only through spoken instructions, this puts the autistic child at a disadvantage. It is in this way that memory can impact executive functioning. As the non-autistic child starts to embed more spoken words and sentences, they will begin forming the ability to embed spoken instructions. These are repeated over their early years and into school, which strengthens their ability to encode, store and retrieve those words (such as speech-based instructions). In this way, their memories build around 'expected' executive functioning skills, such as following spoken instructions and organising themselves. Does that mean autistic children lack the ability to remember and embed? No, it means they are embedding and remembering divergently. An autistic child accessing and recreating musical patterns may develop (or be predisposed to) building connections around these skills, including their memories. Memory can build around any pattern and code, such as speech, written, musical, mathematical, visual composition, etc.

I can use Jay as an example of this. He is deemed deficient in expected EF, yet he can interpret and internally organise musical notes; he can assimilate that information to coordinate his fingers to play music without formal teaching. He can also listen to a pattern of music and recreate it. He seems to do this by mapping the sounds he hears, transferring the audio information to his fingers on the piano, predicting which note is needed, testing his prediction, correcting, and then re-mapping for the correct note. Throughout this, Jay is shifting his attention between the audio and the physical, using his working memory, focusing for 'age-appropriate' periods, and sustaining attention. He also has good fine motor and spatial awareness skills in this task. Jay has heightened EF skills when playing the piano, yet this is not recognised or weighted like EF skills based on spoken instruction.

Jay's ability to follow spoken instructions, organise his school bag, and get himself to the correct room on time are all social organisation skills that need to be embedded often through conversations and spoken reminders. Jay is still working on getting himself ready in the mornings independently; these skills take longer, partly due to his hypermobility and fleeting focus. But Jay's family states that he does not lack focus. Early mornings are often when he is most creative, composing a new piece of music or creating a new coding project. Jay is never shamed for his divergent abilities; his ability to tie his shoelaces or put on his tie will have little bearing on his future. It is great to teach life skills, but expectations placed on autistic children often overlook their whole body and brain divergence.

Many might see Jay's lack of expected EF skills around self-organisation as a flaw, but I see a brilliant musician who learned to play the piano seemingly without external instruction. He is not less skilled; he is just differently skilled. Jay will not embed EF through spoken reminders; he thinks in words, numbers, and sometimes musical notes! Jay will need different support with his EF skills, such as visual, written, or voice note reminders. We need to normalise non-standardised teaching and learning strategies for non-standardised minds.

Standardised tests

'Sometimes the most brilliant and intelligent minds do not shine in standardised tests because they do not have standardised minds.'

Diane Ravitch

Our brains use our past knowledge to make predictions about the world around us. Various factors shape and influence these predictions, including spoken conversations and interactions. For an autistic child, their unique neurosensory profile leads them to construct predictions that may diverge from most non-autistic children. As a result, this can significantly impact the way they respond to standardised questions.

For instance, consider a test question that prompts children to imagine a sunny beach scenario with lots of children playing and laughing. Most children whose past experiences of the beach were not characterised by sensory overload may predict that the children in this scenario would feel excited and happy. However, an autistic child who has encountered sensory overwhelm at a beach due to the sensations of sand and other sensory inputs might have a different prediction. When asked, 'How would you feel running onto that beach?' the autistic child may predict feeling scared or anxious based on their unique sensory experiences. This would not marry with an expected response.

To get a good grade in comprehension and inference tasks, the autistic child cannot use their own reasoning from their own experiences. Instead, they have to guess how a non-autistic child would feel running onto a busy beach. This makes current inference questions deeply flawed for any children and young people who do not experience the world in the 'expected' way, putting these children at a considerable disadvantage.

Autistic children are often assumed to lack inference abilities when, in reality, they could probably predict what another child with a similar neurosensory profile would experience. Still, autistic children often do not get the chance to grow a deep understanding of their own experiences. Autistic children have minimal access to language that describes their own conceptual understanding of the world. A neurosensory divergent autistic child will not often see themselves or their experiences represented in books or TV shows, and I have not heard sensory experiences discussed in many classrooms. Instead, autistic children will hear about 'expected' experiences. When talking about the beach example, a teacher might say, 'Can you imagine how wonderful it would be to run onto the hot sandy beach?' This might contradict an autistic child's own constructed understanding of a beach.

Imagine this the other way around; imagine if non-autistic children had to answer questions based on autistic experiences, but this was not made explicitly clear – so they answered using their own non-autistic inference and conceptual understanding. Let me give you an example inference question:

Billy is in class learning facts about the space programme, which he enjoys. It has been a very long lesson, and Billy has been focusing so intensely on the subject that he has blocked out all the sights and sounds around him. He hasn't noticed that his class has packed up and is lined up for playtime. How do you think Billy feels when the playtime bell rings, signalling that the lesson is over so he can pack up and join the other children outside playing?

A) Billy hears the bell and feels happy that he can go out to play with his friends.

B) The sound of the bell has hurt Billy's ears; he now feels overwhelmed and is rushing to pack up. The sensory stimulation of the classroom overwhelms his senses. Billy's hands are sweaty, and his heart races as he packs up.

Most non-autistic children might identify with A and might reason that this would be Billy's internal thoughts. But as this is a paper based on autistic experiences, they would be marked wrong. Many autistic children might instead identify with B, and they would be marked correct.

Throughout education and life, autistic children are fed non-autistic narratives and corrected when they use their own autistic knowledge of the world. As discussed previously, they might be told, 'That doesn't hurt' when they feel intense pain after banging their leg, or they might be told, 'It is not loud in here' when, for the autistic child, it is extremely loud. Correcting autistic children's experiences and replacing their narratives with non-autistic narratives is confusing for autistic children and fails to validate what they are experiencing.

I was recently observing a speech and language session where a child was asked, 'How would you approach a group of children to ask them to play? Should you say, "Hey, how are you? Can I play with you?" or should you just run up and shout at the group, "Let's play?"' When the child replied with the second option, he was told this was incorrect; he should use the first option! For a child to whom spoken language is challenging, I feel the second option would be absolutely fine and understandable. It made me wonder how this correction might embed in his brain, making him unsure of how to 'correctly' approach a group of children in the future; such conditioning could remove a level of self-assurance in autistic minds.

Autistic conceptual knowledge of the world, their style of communication, learning and socialising are continually questioned and corrected. From having less useful language to describe their experience to having their experiences invalidated by those who do not understand sensory divergence, autistic children have very little chance to embed or demonstrate their own autistic inference.

Sensory access in schools

When autistic children do not consistently access spoken elements of lessons, it becomes crucial to accommodate their preferred learning style and provide instruction in their 'first language.' For some autistic children, video learning, online learning, immersive, hands-on experiences, or learning from books can be more effective. These methods allow them to be fully immersed in the learning process, engaging multiple senses and facilitating a deeper understanding of the subject matter.

Many non-autistic children experience education as an immersive and seamless process where they effortlessly engage with spoken, social, and academic learning. They enter a state of flow, and many can effortlessly embed spoken concepts into their understanding, almost as if learning happens by osmosis. For autistic children, expected conceptual learning may not happen as effortlessly.

Learning does not just happen in the classroom. What children learn throughout their lives plays into their education. Take, for example, a typical weekend walk of a parent and their six-year-old child. For a non-autistic child who accesses speech in the expected way, the experience is a language-rich one. As they stroll through the park, the parent might casually point out the vibrant colours of the flowers, the various animal sounds, and the sweet aroma of freshly cut grass. The child's spoken language development intertwines seamlessly with their environment and experiences. As they encounter a dog playing fetch, the parent might engage the child in a conversation about the dog's breed, its behaviour, and how to approach animals safely. Later, they come across a squirrel darting up a tree, which sparks a discussion about the animal's habits and natural habitat. These interactions, filled with spoken language and verbal exchange, allow the child to effortlessly acquire new vocabulary and grasp abstract concepts.

However, for an autistic child whose speech development differs, this same walk might be experienced through a different lens. The child is walking with their parent, and they are enjoying the feel of the sun on their body, but it is shining brightly into their eyes, so they are shielding their eyes with their hand. The leaves are blowing in the wind and making loud rustling noises. Bird song mingles with the plane noise and cars on the nearby road, and their parent is saying something about a flower. The parent beckons the child over, who looks at the flower; in their mind, they see the words flash 'pink flower' from a book they read the week before. The spoken language this child has picked up is 'pink flower', but they have actually had a sensorily busy experience and will have embedded new concepts from their walk.

When these two children return to school and are asked to write about their weekend, the non-autistic child would be able to draw on all the spoken conversations, whereas the autistic child may not be able to put all their experiences into words. Equally, a child who can access the visual code may have great ideas for their writing but experience challenges expressing their knowledge through speech, or their motor skills might be a barrier to their writing. All these children are developing their conceptual understanding of the world and their capacity to express it in very different ways from one another.

Understanding that there are different neurosensory profiles is hugely important. Although supporting materials may be offered in lessons, such as pictures, PowerPoints and textbooks, our current teaching system is predicated on the idea that the bulk of learning is imparted through knowledgeable teachers speaking from the front of classrooms. Many autistic children are completely unaware that they are experiencing the sensory element within classrooms differently from their non-autistic peers.

Often, neurosensory divergent children have to focus more intensely on accessing lesson information, which can be exhausting. This means these children might be in a high-stress state at school a lot of the time. Autistic children might also become distracted by other sensory inputs and find themselves in trouble for not focusing or for distracting others; they may well feel frustrated and confused about why they find it so hard to access and embed the lesson information. In traditional classroom settings, teachers may not typically receive training regarding the importance of accommodating sensory access via different teaching methods. Nevertheless, as Heidi underscores, this aspect is a critical element in understanding the challenges faced by autistic students within standard classroom instruction.

The way I would receive information... It would be visual if it was written up on the board. A lot of it would be from what was written down or from reading or just thinking about the material in front of me ... my [learning] was very mildly supplemented by listening.

Autistic children need an education that suits their profile. The fact that this is not being offered is not the fault of the child but an issue for society to correct.

Unstructured time in schools

Playgrounds are full of rich and layered social interactions alongside being sensorially busy. Although this can be an enjoyable time, it can also be daunting for autistic children who must navigate the different sensory inputs and social expectations. Without structured, tailored support, autistic children can find these times very challenging.

The playground can be a sensory-rich environment that presents both opportunities and challenges for autistic children. The multitude of sights, sounds, textures, and movements can either overwhelm or captivate their senses. For some autistic children, the cacophony of voices and echoing footsteps might lead to sensory overload, causing them to seek solitude or cover their ears. On the other hand, some may find comfort in being outdoors, such as feeling the cool breeze on their skin or exploring different textures, providing valuable opportunities for sensory exploration and self-regulation. However, it is crucial for educators and peers to be sensitive to individual sensory needs and preferences, allowing autistic children to navigate the playground in ways that support their unique neurosensory profiles. Creating inclusive and sensory-friendly spaces ensures that all children can enjoy the benefits of play while feeling safe and comfortable in their surroundings.

Autistic pupils and other pupils with communication divergence may share a unique understanding of each other's experiences. Research has demonstrated that interactions between children with similar experiences can foster connections, a phenomenon we have observed in the friendships Jay has formed with neurodivergent peers. In these relationships, there appears to be an immediate understanding that Jay doesn't necessarily experience with non-autistic peers. As children mature and communication becomes more complex, this divide can become more noticeable.

Unfortunately, in many school playgrounds, the burden falls on autistic pupils to navigate the complex social world around them. Autistic children are constantly deciphering social cues and codes and cognitively determining how to navigate various social situations. This social curriculum, combined with the academic one, can leave them emotionally and cognitively exhausted. Having spent time processing huge amounts of sensory input from the playground, deciphering social codes and rules, masking and observing during playtimes, they are then asked to settle immediately into lessons. Playtimes are not necessarily the relaxing downtime that they are for other children. This is especially true when children do not have access to activities that are non-speech-based.

For Jay and other autistic children, the desire to connect socially may be profound, but various barriers might hinder them. Many boys play football at lunchtime, but not all boys want to join in or have the motor skills to keep up with their peers. Similarly, lots of girls engage in more layered and complex social groupings, leaving girls with divergent first languages confused as to how to form connections. Enabling connections through different types of activities, such as interest-based clubs and non-speech-based play, can be invaluable.

I saw a wonderful example of this being used in a school recently. The school introduced some building materials and construction play into their Year Three and Four playgrounds. These were items usually found in a reception or nursery playground. There were wooden building blocks and a wooden obstacle course. The group of children who gravitated towards these items were children deemed to have social and emotional and communication differences. The teachers supporting these children found that without the cognitive load of spoken interactions, the children engaged in much more cooperative play and problem-solving.

It is possible to restructure mainstream school environments to be more autism-friendly, but it does take unconventional and innovative thinking from teaching bodies and leadership teams.

School refusal and attachment

When a child's sensory needs and learning requirements are not met in school, it is often the parents who are left to pick up the pieces. As discussed previously, parents often become adept at meeting those needs by sticking to sameness, reducing expectations and allowing the child time to reset. Children who come to feel trauma at school may well avoid school at all costs. When mainstream inclusion is mismanaged, it can lead to autistic pupils feeling excluded, isolated and misunderstood, feelings which are implicated in autistic school refusal.

School environments and staff ethos can make all the difference:

Teaching autistic children requires innovation and a willingness to break away from traditional methods. In Jay's educational journey, one crucial factor has been the ethos of the people around him. Jay's parents have definitely experienced challenges along the way. Some teachers have viewed his need to leave the classroom as a negative adjustment. They have misunderstood his spoken skills as a reflection of his cognitive abilities and have failed to grasp his unique learning profile and potential. In meetings with his mother, descriptions of Jay as disengaged and struggling did not align with the Jay they knew at home. Over the years, it became increasingly evident that the adults who more attuned to his profile and potential achieved better results. Those who supported Jay played a crucial role in shaping outcomes. Interestingly, many of these supportive individuals had direct experience with neurodivergent children or were neurodivergent themselves, which seemed to enhance their empathy and knowledge.

Jay's parents did manage to find a school with a wonderful Head Teacher and Special Educational Needs Coordinator (SENCO), who were committed to supporting him. Inclusion has been front and centre in all the decisions made for him, and his parents were involved at every step of this collaborative process. The most transformative years for Jay have been those when teachers and learning support staff have come up with unconventional ways to engage and support him. These have included friendship supports, whole class sensory time, affirming social stories, motor adjustments for Physical Education lessons and equitable practices such as allowing him to type instead of having to write. Jay has been encouraged to be unapologetically himself, both in school and by his parents at home. Although this sounds idyllic, Jay has experienced sensory and social challenges, and his academic abilities did not always shine through in conventional classrooms.

During lockdown, Jay found it challenging to engage with online learning the way it was being delivered. His parents decided to use a tutor at home. In this quiet, low-arousal environment with 1:1 teaching structured specifically for him, Jay began to realise his full potential – showing abilities we knew were hiding below the surface. When Jay returned to school, his parents requested a dual setting where Jay would be taught some mornings in a low-arousal setting with teacher input. Although this was highly unusual, his school agreed to trial it.

In this dual setting, his 1:1 teacher had high-quality training in supporting autistic children and was able to teach Jay in multimodal ways, which utilised technology so he could learn in an immersive fashion. This suited his learning profile and access requirements. He could consistently access what the teacher was saying because of the quiet environment, and he could learn in enjoyable and engaging ways. The staff at school commented on the positive impact this dual setting had on his ability to engage in lessons. At school, they continued using practices of engaging him through his interests and employing equitable strategies, which have also been pivotal in supporting Jay's learning profile.

I know Jay's parents feel incredibly lucky to have found a school that thinks outside the box and one that saw Jay's potential. Many autistic children, due to the structure of conventional schooling, do not have this opportunity to learn and develop on their own terms. This is not the fault of dedicated teaching staff, but a problem with conventional educational practices and processes currently being followed. Jay is not alone in finding the school environment does not meet all his requirements. Making mainstream schools more autism-friendly and offering dual specialised teaching in low-arousal settings could help support more autistic children to thrive.

Education Health Care Plan (EHCP)

Currently, when a child is identified as autistic and is considered to need educational support other than that offered through a standard mainstream education, they are assessed for an EHCP. This document tends to include targets and supports that help the child catch up with their similarly aged peers and strategies to help them cope in current settings, alongside recommendations on what kind of school a child might need. As demonstrated by Jay's journey, it is evident that autistic children can require a different approach to education, one that is tailored to their primary mode of communication and provides access to low-arousal environments. Unfortunately, without a practical alternative to the conventional school structure centred on standardised goals, many autistic children do not have access to an educational model that effectively addresses their unique learning requirements.

Currently, to show a child has a special educational need, their challenges need to be highlighted in the EHCP, and this can lead to documents which contain deficit-based language to describe autistic children. But there are also many stories of EHCPs being written cooperatively between parents and professionals. An increasing number of professionals recognise the significance of the neurodiversity movement and are aligning their targets accordingly. A friend of mine recently advocated for her child's EHCP to encompass interest-driven supports, monotropism, and the double empathy theory. The possibility of incorporating these concepts into future EHCPs brings hope to many, suggesting that more supportive and affirming services for autistic children may be on the horizon.

For the thousands of EHCPs that *are* issued in a supportive and timely manner, there are many cases where the process is far from supportive. Many children and families face long delays (often years) in being issued with an EHCP. The process of professional assessments and paperwork is long and complex. It can be stressful for parents whose children are struggling within mainstream education and need support as soon as possible. When this is not offered in a timely manner, it can be hugely detrimental to autistic children's well-being.

Central government has tasked councils with the dual purpose of cutting budgets while simultaneously deciding which children are most in need of an EHCP. This can create a 'them and us' situation where boroughs are pitted against parents. There are no winners in this situation. Many families have to go to court against the borough to secure their child's right to access the support provided by an EHCP. People who take council jobs in the SEND department often do so with the hope of helping families but instead find themselves having to cost-cut and reject EHCP applications or go to court to fight against families getting EHCPs. There are numerous advocates whose roles involve assisting families of autistic children in learning SEND law in order to advocate for their child's fundamental right to receive an inclusive education.

For instance, these families may require placement in a special educational needs school, specifically designed to meet the unique requirements of children and young people with special educational needs and disabilities. These schools can be invaluable in providing educational alternatives to mainstream settings. Many parents find these environments better suited to their children's needs due to the availability of tailored education plans and smaller class sizes. However, there is a significant discrepancy between the number of children with EHCP plans or those awaiting plans and the limited availability of special educational needs school places, with fewer than two thousand places available for hundreds of thousands of children in need.

Insufficient availability of Special Educational Needs (SEN) school places often leaves children without appropriate educational options, and there are very few alternatives for children who could access a mainstream curriculum if it were better tailored to their requirements. When no suitable alternatives exist, parents may opt for homeschooling – a challenging but necessary choice. The Children and Families Act 2014 provides legal provisions for educating children when in-school education isn't appropriate, known as Education Other Than At School (EOTAS). However, this process can be even more complex and challenging than attaining an EHCP, and parents regularly have to go to tribunal or to court to justify their reasoning. I know of autistic advocates (who fully understand their child's legal rights to this provision) who have faced huge barriers when attempting to fight for their child's right to an education other than at school. Heidi Mavir is one such advocate who has written candidly about her experiences. She is clear about the many times she and her son experienced hidden bias and ableist assumptions while she fought for the correct education. Heidi now tirelessly advocates for change alongside educating families on finding support through the EOTAS process.[89]

Parents of autistic children should not have to go to court and be pitted against professionals to fight for their child's basic educational needs. These are families already dealing with a huge number of challenges. They are simply seeking answers and support for their children. A suitable education that supports autistic first languages and offers neurodivergent affirming environments would remove many of the barriers families of autistic children currently face. Without these adjustments, autistic children will continue to struggle in the current narrow education system.

---

89   Mavir, H. (2023). Your Child Is Not Broken – Parent Your Neurodivergent Child Without Losing Your Marbles.

PART NINE

TRAUMA

Very few autistic children have not experienced anxiety or trauma. I certainly have never met any. That is an extremely sad statement to write. Autistic children are at increased risk of experiencing trauma, which may stem from the interplay between their sensory profile and their environment, as well as from challenging social interactions.

Sensory trauma

Sensory trauma profoundly affects autistic children when they encounter overwhelming or distressing sensory stimuli, disrupting the regulation of their nervous systems. This can result from any environment or experience where they might experience sensory overload. As discussed previously, sensory input that seems unremarkable to non-autistic people can be excruciating for autistic children. There can also be an accumulative effect when autistic children are exposed to sensorily busy environments on an ongoing basis. Sensory trauma may also trigger anxiety and hypervigilance.

I liken this to a metaphorical sensory tightrope, where the land they have to step off represents familiar safety (such as a home), and the tightrope represents potential sensory trauma (busy environments). Imagine an autistic child stepping off that precipice every day, tentatively walking out onto that tightrope with the potential they could fall at any moment. There could be a change to routine, a fire alarm test, a new child in the class, a change to a classroom, a social falling out, or an instance of being told off; there are so many moments when an autistic child might experience both small and large traumas throughout the day.

If anxiety related to sensory divergence becomes too intense, it can manifest as extreme behaviours such as Obsessive Compulsive Disorder, where a person feels they must control their environment in order to feel safe, or eating disorders, where the underlying reason can be sensory aversions or a need to control.

Things can be done to mitigate sensory trauma. Understanding and validating the daily experiences of autistic children is a good starting point.

Identity rejection and trauma

I guess neurodivergent children were judged, and it's hard for me to pinpoint exactly how, but I just have a lot of emotional memories of feeling like people weren't that nice and that it was kind of difficult just going day-to-day and because I wasn't the kind of person that was happy being on my own or cutting myself off... I kind of needed people but found them really difficult, and they did not seem to like my personality. So it was like a kind of horrible irony of my character.

(Jules, autistic adult)

Jules puts the rejection she felt down to her own character. Sadly, this is how many autistic children and adults feel like there is something inherently wrong with them. Here, I want to discuss a new term which is being used: Rejection Sensitivity Dysphoria. This describes people who are overly sensitive to rejection. I would like to be very clear here. I do not believe that autistic people are 'more' sensitive to rejection.

Autistic children experience more episodes of rejection than most children, and they inevitably notice a pattern of rejection. Others can misinterpret their style of communication as being offensive. Their responses to sensory trauma are often misunderstood. They are expected to change their natural ways of being and catch up with expected developmental milestones, and they are expected to thrive in settings and systems not built around their requirements. This identity rejection permeates through every part of their lives. If this life sounds untenable, that is because it is.

People used to laugh at me all the time for things I did and said that was just me being me .... and my 'friends' would literally crack up over certain things I did unintentionally (so they were laughing at me for sure).

(Heidi, autistic adult)

Although autistic children are part of school communities, many are ostracised by mainly non-autistic social groups. Instead, they exist on the periphery because of the divide between autistic communication and interests and non-autistic communication and interests.

Autistic children are often positioned as outsiders who need to change to be less of everything they naturally are in order to fit in. Less noisy, less bouncy, less abrasive, less picky, less anxious, less insular, less frustrated – really, less different from the expected way of being. Behaviour policies often do not take into account the way autistic children experience school and how these experiences might impact behaviour. When rejection and correction become too much, autistic children may behave in ways that challenge others and may be reprimanded for their behaviour. When autistic children are reprimanded for such behaviour, it does little to help them and only serves to invalidate their experiences further. Negative reinforcements only add to their trauma.

If neurodivergent and autistic children's names consistently appear on the negative side of behaviour charts, it should flag an issue within the environment rather than something inherent within those children. More comprehensive support may be necessary. Behaviour charts are actually quite disempowering. Imagine if you had a behaviour chart in your workplace and every day your name was on the negative list. Would that feel motivational? Behaviour charts often work for children who are following standardised developmental trajectories and who can adhere to expected rules. In other children, these systems can instil a sense of fear, failure and perfectionism.

Living life this way can leave the autistic child in a state of fear that they are getting life wrong. When trying to fit in, they might try to change themselves to appear more like non-autistic people. This is called masking and involves lots of effort and internal, often subconscious, practice at blending in. So, when a child who is masking puts a foot wrong, they feel like all their effort was wasted. The disappointment in themselves is huge. Failed friendships are devastating – because they fought so hard to get those friendships.

Autistic children are constantly policing themselves internally and are often being policed externally, which means many exist in a social trauma state. They can become anxious in social situations because it has been reinforced through past interactions that they often say or do the 'wrong' thing. When they are rejected, it is on top of lots of previous social and emotional rejections.

Jules, an autistic adult, explains how she felt about social interactions at school:

> *I knew I couldn't manage social conversations with people who I knew quite well but weren't my friends... so I would go and hide in the classroom.*

Heidi, an autistic adult, also experienced social anxiety as a child:

> *I thought everyone did this. And this is what life looked like: you'd go to school highly anxious, worrying about every social encounter.*

Autistic children who attempt to fit in with group dynamics and hidden social rules can find this exhausting, which can impact their mental health. When they do find a friend or a group who accepts them as they are, they can feel intensely happy and connected.

Finding my people was so hard at school – I often felt lonely but also felt shame about having no friends. I pretended to teachers and to my parents that I was fine in school, but really, kids were so unkind to me. I managed to get one friend who also got bullied, and we stuck to each other like glue. One of my greatest joys as I've gotten older has been discovering friends who accept me just as I am.

(Millie, autistic adult)

Chronic Masking

I have called autistic masking *chronic masking*. Chronic masking is unlike everyday situations where someone might present a certain aspect of their personality, such as being more professional at work or being more laid back with certain friends. Autistic masking is likely to come about for many different reasons. As many autistic children learn social concepts and behaviour expectations later than their peers, they may find themselves 'being corrected' many times with very little understanding of why they are being corrected. This negative feedback can have a detrimental effect on autistic children.

Positive feedback in childhood helps a child to develop a strong sense of self; when a child is constantly reassured that their traits and ways of being in the world are accepted and celebrated, that child learns that *they* are accepted and celebrated. Autistic childhood traits are often not so readily rewarded. Parents and teachers caring for a child who does not follow an 'expected' path may critique unexpected behaviours and attempt to correct that child to follow 'expected' behaviours. Autistic children can then grow up in a state of heightened vigilance or perfectionism, where they attempt to follow the rules for 'correct' behaviour.

For autistic children, rules can become very important as they attempt to navigate this world of social and behavioural expectations. Only these rules are not hard and fast. For example, you can joke with your friends in the playground, but you can't when you are lining up for a class photo. In the classroom, you definitely cannot joke with your friends, except when the teacher says it is okay because the teacher has made a joke. This can be confusing for autistic children who are trying to follow rules that have not necessarily been seamlessly embedded through conversations. Autistic children are often attempting to embed rules as they are corrected. As you can imagine, this is a stressful endeavour.

Autistic children also mask in social situations. Many autistic children access spoken language in a gestalt manner, meaning they copy chunks of communication and apply that to different contexts. They may appear socially awkward for this reason. When they do use their own style of communication, they might be rejected for seeming unusual. Autistic children also develop their social likes and dislikes along their own developmental timelines and pathways, meaning their interests might not appeal to similarly aged non-autistic children. Identity rejection by others is confusing for autistic children. They are just being themselves and looking for friendship and acceptance from their peers. Many autistic children learn the skill of pretending to like the things that non-autistic children like and to speak in the same way as non-autistic children. In this way, they can find acceptance in non-autistic groups.

Even with other autistic and neurodivergent children, the skill of being a friend presents challenges for some autistic children. Some autistic children's communication is very direct, and this can lead to social misunderstandings. For example, when Jay's friend recently became class captain, Jay told his friend that he was not happy as Jay wanted to be class captain, and this upset Jay's friend very much. Jay did not want to hurt his friend's feelings and explained he was only being honest. Attempting to teach an autistic child that sometimes lying is a nice thing to do is complex. Even lying to save another person's feelings is a type of masking because it is not a natural trait for many autistic children. It is important to state here Jay would never intentionally hurt someone else's feelings. Autistic communication is often misunderstood as rude or unkind when, in reality, it is just honest and straightforward.

Living under a cloud of identity rejection is to feel that no part of you is accepted. Maslow's hierarchy of needs is a model which explains human needs. Maslow places physiological needs as the most important of our human needs, followed by safety, then love and belonging. The model states that feelings of safety and belonging are necessary before a person can achieve self-esteem and self-actualisation. This feeling of belonging does not have to come from similarly aged peers. It can come from anywhere: family, grandparents, online friends, even animals. There is a wonderful autistic young person called Summer Farrelly who advocates for finding belonging with chickens and dogs. They state that they found it too difficult to maintain autistic to non-autistic relationships and was often bullied, but with animals they felt safe as they knew animals would not judge them or be unkind.[90]

While non-autistic individuals might find the concept of completely concealing oneself unfamiliar, it is presently a necessary part of many autistic lives. Unmasking, the process through which a person exhibits more natural autistic traits, can carry significant risks in social interactions. Autistic children who do not or cannot mask can be vulnerable to judgment from others in society. TJ is an American autistic writer[91] who explores the experience of being black and autistic. She advises her children that autistic individuals often face a choice

90   Autistic Perspectives - Summer Farrelly. (2021). ABOUT CHICKENS TO LOVE. [online] Available at: https://summerfarrelly.com.au/animal-assisted-learning/ [Accessed 26 Aug. 2023].

91   www.instagram.com. Tiffany Joseph. Instagram. [online] Available at: https://www.instagram.com/p/CciuYa0uDut/?utm_source=ig_web_copy_link&igshid=MzRlODBiNWFlZA== [Accessed 26 Aug. 2023].

between engaging in behaviours that make *them* feel comfortable versus behaviours that put others at ease. She explains that when others are uncomfortable or challenged, their reactions may range from confusion and fear to anger and frustration. Consequently, at times, opting to make others feel comfortable by masking can be a safer course of action. Although TJ acknowledges this is an unfair request, it is often necessary.

In many instances, masking is not a conscious choice; it arises from the need to 'fit in' and conform to societal norms to maintain autistic safety.

It's exhausting to be in a perpetual state of striving to do things 'correctly' while being uncertain about what that entails.

(Leah, autistic child)

Meltdowns and Shutdowns

Having concentrated hubs that take in lots of information means there are multiple ways an autistic child's brain might become overloaded. The most obvious traits associated with overloaded neurological systems are meltdowns or shutdowns. In a meltdown, it is clear to see the child's distress; they may end up shouting, throwing things, or lashing out.

Shutdowns are similar to meltdowns, but the child's

system simply cuts out. On the surface, they may look calm, but internally their heart may race, their palms may be sweaty, they may lose their ability to speak, and they may feel frozen and in a fearful state. Autistic children have told me that a shutdown feels like being trapped inside a burning building. Your brain just stops working; it feels like you cannot move or speak. You want whatever is happening to stop, but you cannot stop it. All your usual coping strategies and abilities just cease to be available. It is almost like the overload knocks out a whole hub of brain connectivity, like a blown fuse in the brain, but it doesn't stop the sensory input from their environment; they still feel all the overload and trauma but cannot express what is happening to them. Their ability to think clearly may be impacted, and other sensory systems may become heightened. On the outside, the child may seem quiet, vacant, and even calm; however, internally, this state is like being trapped in a cacophony of internal processes.

It may be helpful to think of a child's response in shutdown or meltdown as being entirely out of their control. Meltdowns and shutdowns are almost like a conscious fit, where the child's overloaded brain is a mass of electrical and chemical signals that filter down into their bodily reactions. Jordan James (previously Joe James) is an autistic advocate who describes his meltdowns in exactly this way. Jordan says that he used to feel huge regret after any meltdown but he has come to understand that being in a state of overload is a neurological and biological reaction that is hard to override. It is obviously inappropriate to judge a child for losing control of their body when they have an epileptic fit. Autistic children in overload have a similar experience and need to be supported just as one would support any child in distress. It is scary and exhausting for the child.

This is where behaviourist approaches can be hugely counterproductive. Teaching autistic children to suppress or ignore their internal processes in an attempt to reduce behaviours does not address their needs and can be detrimental. Instead, this approach often leads autistic children to mask their natural response to stress, further disconnecting from their own sensory experiences. This suppression is akin to shaking a Coke bottle throughout the day, with the child trying to keep a lid on their emotions and challenges at school or nursery. Being in this state can mean that small stressors can have a cumulative effect, tipping children into an uncontrollable overload or shutdown. Many parents report that schools tell them that their child is 'fine in school'; their autistic child seems to 'save up' these intense reactions for when they return home, where they feel safe to unmask and release the stresses of the day. Many autistic behaviours perceived as challenging may arise from the constant struggle autistic children face in navigating a world that is not built around their requirements.

In school, there can be all kinds of different experiences which can trigger overload. When autistic children experience too much sensory information or when they access information that is hard to process, they can become overloaded. For example, when their brain has predicted what will happen next and instead, something unexpected happens, this information does not marry with their pre-existing concepts: it can feel like a glitch in their system. Their brain requires them to forge a new pathway of conceptual understanding.

New conceptual pathways are much harder to form and take time to embed. This might happen when, for example, the school routine changes: the autistic child may have built strong conceptual and sensory connections to their routine and changes to this must be embedded beforehand to help them build up their conceptual understanding. When a child finds it hard to process information that does not sit well with their current understanding of the world, they often get stuck in a loop of trying to fix the unfixable 'glitch'. It can seem like they are running the event back in their head in the way it was 'supposed to happen'; all this neurological activity can result in overload.

An autistic child may be unable to tell you what has triggered their stress response, and they may not know themselves. It can be the result of a cumulative effect, or it can be from something they have not yet processed or from something they did not fully understand. When you ask an autistic child about their experiences, their answer may be much more complex than a non-autistic child's, but they may not have the tools or language to express this complexity. For example, a teacher may ask if they had a good playtime; an autistic child's playtime experience could include many of the above triggers but may also include fun and happy moments. Therefore, their answer may be, 'It was good,' or, 'I don't know,' neither of which reveals much about how their playtime actually was.

Both meltdowns and shutdowns are uncontrollable mental responses to overload. Just as with an overloaded electrical circuit, very little can be done once the overload starts. The only course of action is often to unplug. In autistic children, this might look like removing and lowering sensory inputs, reducing expectations, and having a safe space where they can retreat. Meltdowns and shutdowns are emotionally and physically exhausting, and autistic children need empathy and support in these moments. I have consistently found that validating what they are experiencing and reassurance during and after episodes can help calm children. Meltdowns and shutdowns come about through stress, anxiety and frustration, so the aim is always to reduce the stressors on the child.

Burnout

Some autistic children are in a constant state of sensory overload, masking, internal confusion and feigning self-regulation. Being in this state for a prolonged period of time means their brain is constantly 'on' with electrical impulses and chemicals being triggered in the autistic child's body and brain. This can lead to something called burnout, where the brain effectively blows a fuse and stops working.

Burnout is a state some autistic children find themselves in when the demands placed on them (which are often not appropriate for their profile) overwhelm them. Burnout is a physical and mental health crisis which needs to be taken seriously. A child who is forced to push through burnout is likely to spiral into a more serious mental health crisis.

Psychological Therapy

Traditional talking therapy may not be suitable for autistic children as it is based on talking, which is not all autistic children's preferred form of communication. It is also possible that non-autistic therapists may not be able to empathise fully with autistic experiences. Cognitive Behavioural Therapy (CBT) might be offered, but this concentrates on changing thought patterns and may not address broader societal issues or sensory trauma. It could teach autistic children to further suppress their discomfort in a bid to rid themselves of negative thought patterns.

Positive outcomes have emerged from teaching autistic children relaxation techniques. I've witnessed the effectiveness of art, music, and play therapy, especially when it focuses on interactive play or artistic expression of their emotions (not instruction on how to play). Future support for autistic children should prioritise trauma reduction, validation of their experiences, and enhancing access.

Other therapies offered to autistic children

Up until recently, the aim of therapy for autistic children has been to help them reach non-autistic milestones or to help them reduce their autistic traits. These aims are not about validating autistic sensory and motor experiences or reducing autistic trauma.

There has been a growing recognition that these approaches are not in the best interest of autistic children. Therefore, parents need to be aware of the type of therapy they are choosing for their child. A register of neurodiversity-affirming therapists could prove very useful in this regard.

There are certainly therapists who focus on nurturing autistic skills, reducing trauma and using autistic interests and preferred communication to engage them.

Radical acceptance of autistic traits means watching to see how their traits are serving them rather than attempting to alter autistic traits to align with what serves non-autistic children. Were autistic children to be afforded equity and understanding in our society, therapies could also focus on assisting them to unmask safely.

PART TEN:
A MANIFESTO FOR CHANGE

Many years ago, before I was a teacher, I worked as a process manager. The lessons I learned from that experience are highly relevant to the current challenges in moving the autism narrative forward. In my role, I would assess departments, map out their processes in flow charts, and identify any counterproductive practices. When questioning the reasons behind certain processes, I often encountered the response, 'It's just how it's always been done.' Many people had become so accustomed to these methods that they could not see alternatives. Brainstorming new and improved processes was eye-opening for all concerned, but I often faced resistance when implementing these changes as it required unlearning old ways and adapting to new ones, which many found cognitively and emotionally challenging.

We now face a similar need for change regarding autism. Our current processes and procedures do not support autistic children effectively. Conventional knowledge, developmental rules, and expectations are at odds with the route autistic children take. Our medical, educational and societal systems are based on non-autistic sensory experiences of the world. If systems were designed around autistic requirements, the average child's experience might align more closely with autism, and the benchmarks for development and education would be tailored to *their* needs. This approach might embrace interest-driven education based on exploratory investigation and interests, and would also recognise the paramount importance of sensory access.

Listening to the experiences of autistic adults, advocates, parents and professionals who reject conventional knowledge and embrace autistic children's requirements, it is obvious that autistic children thrive when they are allowed to be themselves and are supported by an accepting and equitable environment. Kristy Forbes is a wonderful autistic advocate who teaches just this; I have learned so much from her narrative of radical acceptance – the process of not controlling, judging or invalidating children's natural ways of being. Radical acceptance means viewing autistic traits not as problematic behaviours but as unique characteristics that deserve respect and understanding. Providing co-regulating supports and sensory-friendly environments empowers autistic children to flourish as their authentic selves.

A shift towards a more equitable life for autistic children would require a comprehensive transformation in societal attitudes. This could lead to changes in the policies governing autistic children, as well as reforms in the diagnosis process and in the type of support they receive. By mapping a new suggested pathway from birth to adulthood[92]* and framing autism through a neurosensory divergent lens, we could empower autistic children to thrive in a world that celebrates and values their unique contributions.

A road map for the future

Birth and parenthood:

To ensure a comprehensive and empathetic approach to birth and parenthood, it is vital to involve autistic individuals and parents in developing resources. Parenting an autistic baby can bring joy and challenges, much like any baby. However, babies and toddlers with divergent neurosensory profiles may present unique complexities in sleep, feeding, and potty training. Providing parents access to various lived experience accounts could be invaluable in understanding their child's journey. Resources should avoid deficit-based models and empower parents to make informed choices that align with their child's profile.

A wealth of knowledge from both autistic individuals

---

92   * This is by no means an exhaustive list but does include suggestions to prompt further discussion.

and parents of autistic babies already exists. Collating such expertise alongside input from professionals could yield comprehensive documents that serve as practical guides. Mapping babies' sensory profiles and divergent language development early on could lead to more tailored and individualised support strategies, promoting optimal development and well-being from the earliest stages of life.

Autistic-led research into supports:

Research which informs autistic diagnosis, therapies, support and education should take an inside-out approach. Autistic children experience the world in ways that differ tangibly from their non-autistic peers. More research into sensory profiles, divergent pattern spotting and motor divergence could help to better explain autistic developmental trajectories.

To support and understand autistic perspectives, being inquisitive about experiences is essential. By actively listening to autistic children and adults, society can gain invaluable insights and make more informed decisions regarding education and support. Autistic-led research may offer the most comprehensive inside-out approach, while collaborative research, which includes autistic participants as co-researchers, could also prove invaluable.

Diagnosis:

The diagnostic approach should shift from solely focusing on mapping behaviours to a more comprehensive understanding of internal processes, including sensory profiles.

Diagnostic profiles could encompass the following:

- Sensory profiling
- Divergent pattern recognition profile
- Spoken communication mapping
- The autistic child's first language mapping
- Testing for sensory abundance and deprivation, to include child and parental reports
- Monotropic and interest-driven learning profile
- Motor development mapping
- Identification of common co-occurring conditions warranting further investigation

This shift in approach is crucial for providing targeted and practical support tailored to each autistic child's unique profile.

Educational support documents such as EHCPs

These documents should recognise and value the unique developmental trajectory of each autistic child, focusing on their neurosensory profile and possible motor divergence. Along with identifying each child's sensory access to learning, their preferred communication and their optimal learning environment.

Social and Emotional:

- Social targets to be based on a child's language acquisition
- Autistic children to have a programme of learning about their own sensory profile (to assist children in self-advocacy for their sensory requirements)
- Social support to be documented for unstructured times

Environments:

- All autistic children to have continual access to low-arousal settings
- All autistic children to have access to an ND support person/ co-regulator in school
- All autistic children to have sensory regulation days in their plan where they can reset or work from home when needed
- Documented advice for when a child requires a different setting to mainstream or a dual setting

Learning:

- Interest-driven educational opportunities to be documented
- Multi-sensory resources to be developed to support EF and in-class learning
- Motor targets to take into account a child's disability and to list necessary adjustments

Communication:

- Targets to be developed that value non speech-based play
- Targets to be developed that value different types of communication
- Support staff to help in mapping a child's pattern spotting and first language
- Communication scaffolding to be offered in a low-arousal setting
- AAC (augmentative and alternative communication) and innovative communication strategies to be explored as an immersive language learning experience

Training and therapy:

- Plans to document the requirement for whole school community training on autistic communication, sensory access to learning, sensory profiles, inclusive social practices and co-regulation strategies
- All therapies to be neuro and sensory diversity-affirming

EHCPs should not be drafted by the people who decide on funding because of the potential conflict of interest. Education support documents should always document the true educational requirements of a child. It needs to be acknowledged that mainstream schooling is not always optimal for autistic children, and major adjustments should be implemented to offer autistic children equity in education. The practice of families having to go to court to access EHCPs or other supports needs to cease. This is a practice that hurts neurodivergent families.

To create genuinely inclusive Education Support documents such as EHCPs, there should be equal collaboration with parents, caregivers, and children to seek their insights and their understanding of strengths, challenges, and preferences.

EYFS / National Curriculum and standardised targets

To provide equity for autistic children, it is vital to provide opportunities based on their profile rather than their age. This means moving away from standardised targets. It may be the case that to provide true equity, autistic children would benefit from schools that are not based on age-related targets and instead incorporate self-directed learning.

Inclusive education could encompass self-directed learning as an integral part of their offering. Recognising that traditional teaching methods may not suit all autistic children, schools could embrace flexible and individualised approaches that cater to their unique learning styles and preferences.

Learning profiles:

Divergent learning profiles (spiky profiles) should be recognised and accommodated. This includes support for children who can perform well academically in low-arousal settings but face challenges in demonstrating their abilities at school. This could mean offering dual settings to more children.

We must also investigate and provide sensory access to teaching resources through multi-modal approaches, ensuring that all students can fully engage with the learning materials. Moreover, it is essential to document and celebrate spiky profiles, highlighting a child's talents and abilities in various areas. We should extend this celebration beyond academic achievements and include any unexpected abilities that fall outside the traditional academic skills.

Tests:

Tests should be revised to remove questions that focus solely on non-autistic lived experiences for autistic children. When designing tests, we must consider the individual's spoken communication levels and consider alternative forms of testing, such as multi-modal assessments, which may be more suitable and accommodating for many autistic children. By ensuring tests are inclusive and tailored to the diverse needs of all learners, we can promote a fair and accurate evaluation of their abilities and knowledge.

Positive language:

The use of words such as delay, deficit, or disorder is not helpful when describing autistic children. There is more on this on my website under the Positive Language Project.

Using positive language to describe autistic individuals does not negate the challenges autistic children face. Autism presents in many ways as a disability. Neurological, sensory and motor divergence impacts individuals to varying degrees, potentially causing more significant challenges for some than for others. This can be acknowledged without using deficit-based language.

Inclusive and validating therapy:

Therapeutic approaches for autistic children should be tailored to foster a deeper understanding and acceptance of their distinctive profiles. The integration of co-regulation strategies is essential. The central objective of therapy should revolve around dismantling sensory, motor, and social obstacles that could impede the child's growth and overall welfare. This should involve scaffolding skills while validating autistic developmental trajectories.

Autistic play:

We should embrace and celebrate autistic play in all its forms. Every style of play, including investigative non speech-based play, should be encouraged and supported. It is essential to create a safe environment where autistic children can explore and investigate through various sensory experiences without judgement. Being inquisitive about unexpected investigative play can yield valuable knowledge and insights. It is useful to understand that non-speech-based play is a fundamental and meaningful stage of development for autistic children.

Sensory aids:

Professionals should actively explore the implementation of sensory aids, such as auditory and visual supports, to cater to the individual needs of autistic children. For instance, incorporating listening devices in the classroom can improve learning for those who require enhanced auditory access.

More research is needed to identify and create innovative aids that can significantly enhance the quality of life for autistic children. By investing in the exploration of new technologies and strategies, we can better understand the specific requirements of each child and tailor interventions to provide the most effective sensory support.

Sensory necessary adjustments:

Alongside aids, we can make easy adjustments to help autistic children with their sensory requirements. Below, I list just a few ideas. A more comprehensive list is available on my website.

- Autistic-friendly uniforms to alleviate distressing

tactile sensory experiences

- Sensory aids to be available for any student that needs them
- Sensory access supports and multi-modal resources
- Out-of-class pass and support staff to be available
- Continual access to low-arousal environments

It should be acknowledged that sensory divergence can change. Therefore, a child's requirement for adjustments is dynamic, and staff supporting autistic children should be aware of this.

Although some of these adjustments may seem difficult to implement, it needs to be accepted that this is not the fault of the autistic child. Therefore, if they become overwhelmed in an environment that is not meeting their sensory requirements, it should be noted that the environment is inappropriate, not the child.

Sensory Environments: Creating supportive settings

In-school supports like soft lighting, reduced visual clutter, and sensory tools like fidget toys or noise-cancelling headphones are helpful. However, in-classroom support may not always be sufficient to regulate sensory responses and reduce sensory trauma.

School settings could be improved through a collaborative consultation process between autistic people, affirming autistic researchers and school leadership teams. Through widespread consultations, leadership teams could look to implement robust environmental sensory solutions within schools.

Autistic requirement for unplugging:

Autistic children often require 'unplugging' from sensory input due to their heightened sensitivity. What may seem ordinary or unremarkable to non-autistic children can be overwhelming for autistic children, leading to sensory overload and increased stress. To address this need, we must create safe and supportive spaces where autistic children can take a break and regulate their sensory experiences. These designated areas should be free from excessive sensory stimuli, providing a calm and quiet environment. By recognising and respecting their need to 'unplug', we can help prevent sensory overload and reduce anxiety, allowing autistic children to recharge and feel more comfortable in their surroundings.

Autistic requirement for movement and stimming:

Incorporating movement and stimming activities should be integral to an autistic child's daily routine. These activities regulate their sensory system and promote their overall well-being. To encourage inclusive practices, some movement-based activities could be done as whole-class activities, fostering a sense of belonging and understanding among all students.

Schools should collaborate closely with parents to provide support when autistic children become overwhelmed at school, leading to behaviours that challenge at home. This collaborative approach ensures that the child's well-being is prioritised at school and at home, contributing to their overall success and happiness.

Equitable behaviour strategies:

Behaviour strategies where children are compared based on their behaviour or contributions can be damaging to autistic and neurodivergent children unless they are offered equity in such systems. This is because adhering to expected behaviour, self-organisation, focus and communication targets can be at odds with autistic profiles.

Autistic communication:

Autistic communication is diverse and multifaceted. It is important we recognise that each autistic child may have their own unique first language. While speech-based communication works well for many, it may not be the most effective means for neurosensory divergent (NSD) autistic children. It is essential to prioritise and support their preferred forms of communication, which may include non-verbal methods such as augmentative and alternative communication (AAC), sign language, picture based and written communication and musical or tactile-based communication.

Autistic body communication is a valid and essential means by which some autistic children express their wants and needs. It should be respected and valued, as it often serves as their primary mode of communication.

Practitioners and teachers should understand that autistic communication can sometimes sound harsh and direct, especially when children feel overwhelmed. It is important to ascertain the intention behind autistic communication and to be mindful that sensory barriers to speech can result in a more direct style. Speech can also be effortful, so autistic children may need adjustments in group or class discussions.

By reducing and scaffolding speech-based expectations, we create an inclusive and supportive environment where autistic children can express themselves fully and comfortably. Embracing and validating their diverse ways of communicating empowers autistic children to actively participate in their social and educational experiences.

Subject think and info dumping:

Subject think and info dumping should be considered accepted forms of communication. Teaching non-autistic children about info dumping can help them understand and appreciate the depth of knowledge and passion that autistic children have for their particular interests. Educators can play a pivotal role in facilitating these interactions by promoting a culture of acceptance and appreciation for diverse interests and communication styles.

Interests:

Autistic children's intense and passionate special interests are a window into their unique ways of learning and engaging with the world. By incorporating their special interests into their education, we can tap into their intrinsic motivation, making the learning experience more enjoyable and meaningful for them. When we validate and support their passions, we empower autistic children to excel in areas that genuinely captivate their curiosity and potential. This approach fosters a positive learning environment where their strengths are celebrated and nurtured, leading to greater self-worth and accomplishment.

Teaching about autistic experiences:

To promote a deeper understanding of autistic inference and sensory experiences, we must incorporate a diverse range of autistic perspectives into the curriculum, including books and resources written by autistic authors.

By providing these resources, we empower autistic children to better understand and express their own sensory experiences. Simultaneously, non-autistic children can gain valuable insights into the unique perspectives of their autistic peers, fostering empathy and acceptance.

Autistic need for routine:

The autistic need for sameness should be viewed as a coping mechanism used to reduce the possibility of social or sensory trauma. For some autistic individuals, familiar and predictable routines provide comfort and security in an overwhelming world. Affirming social stories which help with transitions and changes should be used.

Some autistic children need flexible routines. Allowing autistic children to have input, choices and autonomy over their own routines offers autistic children equity through a collaborative approach.

Social barriers and identity rejection:

It is useful to recognise that communication and social barriers exist between autistic and non-autistic individuals. Promoting inclusive social interactions is critical to creating a supportive and accepting school community. Educating children about neurodiversity and NSD autism could help to build empathy and understanding, cultivating an environment where differences are celebrated. Organising inclusive activities that encourage diverse social interactions allows students to connect on various levels, fostering meaningful relationships and friendships and reducing the autistic requirement to mask.

Providing opportunities for non-speech-based play means we can ensure a well-rounded and inclusive educational experience. Implementing whole-school teaching on inclusive and equitable playground expectations ensures that all students can engage in play comfortably and without judgement.

Encouraging self-advocacy:

Empowering autistic children with self-advocacy skills is essential for fostering their autonomy and confidence. By encouraging them to articulate their needs and preferences, we give them a sense of agency over their lives and reduce the need to mask. Teaching self-advocacy helps them identify the support they require to thrive and to navigate any challenges they may encounter. This active involvement in their education and well-being allows them to play an integral role in shaping their own developmental journey. As adults, they will be better equipped to communicate effectively with others, seek appropriate accommodations, and advocate for their rights.

Psychological therapy:

Psychological therapy for autistic children and young individuals should acknowledge the disparity between their present experiences and their envisioned lives, where their sensory needs receive full support, and their distinctive identities are both respected and embraced by adults and peers alike. This therapeutic approach should serve as a bridge across this divide, offering the essential support, tools, and strategies required to navigate the challenges inherent in a world not built around their requirements. Additionally, therapy should actively foster the development of robust self-awareness and self-acceptance, equipping them with the confidence to advocate for their preferences and requirements effectively.

Pathways:

Autistic children deserve access to the same opportunities and future aspirations as non-autistic children. The fact a child is autistic and has sensory access requirements should not prevent them from having those opportunities. To deny access to a disabled person on the basis of their disability is discrimination. There needs to be many more resources that discuss autistic futures with positivity.

Families:

Many families of autistic children feel isolated. They are often not as much part of wider school communities. Autistic families would benefit greatly from more spaces and environments that are welcoming and with tailored elements that meet autistic requirements. This includes autism-friendly after-school clubs alongside inclusive social events. This is something which is lacking in many communities.

Whole communities:

Parents can face stigma and incorrect assumptions when they reveal their child is autistic. Promoting understanding that autism is a sensory, neurological and/or motor divergence could go some way to removing that stigma. Autistic children whose basic needs are met and whose autistic communication is valued and validated will feel more self-assured. Changing societal attitudes towards autistic children is crucial in creating a more inclusive and empathetic world. It requires us to challenge stereotypes and misconceptions about autism and promote a deeper understanding of diversity.

Instead of viewing autism as a deficit, society should recognise the unique strengths and talents that autistic children possess. By actively involving autistic adults, children and their families in advocacy and decision-making processes, we can ensure their voices are heard and respected. Providing the necessary support and accommodations will enable autistic children to thrive. Ultimately, changing societal attitudes involves creating a world where every child is accepted and celebrated for who they are.

Where are we going?

I opened this book with the idea that this is the fight song of so many people. There is not one person involved in an autistic child's life that *wants* to fight for autistic basic needs and rights to be met. Everyone wants a cohesive process where autistic profiles are understood and supported.

By showing where we are now and how we got here, my hope is that this book goes some way to dismantling many outdated beliefs. Elevating the significance of sensory access and prioritising autistic first languages highlights the need for policies and procedures to be adapted to meet autistic children's requirements. This includes reducing sensory trauma and identity rejection. Autistic children and families cannot affect change in any of these areas; they are not at fault and never were. For so long, autistic profiles have been misunderstood.

Neurosensory Divergence asks that we step away from a deficit-based model where the aim is to change autistic behaviours and instead take an inside-out approach. All autistic people have different life experiences, which are all valid and important. Neurosensory Divergence is a part of that story. To ensure society fully understands what is needed, autistic voices should be listened to above all else.

This is not a book about autism awareness or acceptance. It is about the people around autistic children committing to creating an equitable life for every single autistic child. There *is* another way; a new road map to follow. This is where we are going.

WORK WITH ME

To find out more about Helen's work to bring about positive change for autistic and neurodivergent children, you can go to her website or follow her on her socials.

Website
www.outsidetheboxsensory.com

Socials
Instagram
@otbsensory

Facebook
@OTBSensory
@HelenDanielNDSupport

You can find out more about how to book Helen to speak for your organisation by emailing:

hello@outsidetheboxsensory.com